Advanced Nursing Skills
Principles and Practice

Typeset by
Saxon Graphics Ltd., Derby

Printed in the UK by the Alden Group, Oxford

Advanced Nursing Skills
Principles and Practice

Molly Courtenay

PhD, MSc, BSc, RGN, RNT, Cert Ed

Independent Consultant and Honorary Visiting Fellow
Department of Professional Education in Community Studies
The University of Reading

CONTENTS

Chapter 5

Chapter 6

Chapter 7

Chapter 8

Appendix 1:

PREFACE

The initiative for the development of this book arose from the production of a series of distance learning packages designed to examine a number of advanced nursing skills. The learning packages were designed for nurses working in one Hospital Trust who had expanded their roles into a number of different clinical areas. At the time of the development of the packages, the Assistant Director of Nursing was concerned that her nursing staff were increasingly becoming involved in practical skills previously seen as medical territory, but lacked the necessary knowledge to make the professional decisions they were frequently required to make. Therefore, a central aim of the packages was to provide staff with the knowledge underpinning the practical skills in which they were involved, enabling them to exercise the professional judgements expected of them in the practice setting. The distance learning material that was eventually developed was positively received and has since been circulated and used in a number of hospital trusts.

Although there is coverage of some areas of expanded practice in some of the nursing journals, there would appear to be few books available examining these advanced nursing skills. Therefore, it was decided to develop the distance learning material into a book.

The author has attempted to bring together widely available information into a single, easy to use, practice-based text. It should not be used in isolation but in conjunction with local policies and guidelines. It is hoped, that by identifying the knowledge base which underpins each of the advanced nursing skills described, along with the research evidence upon which each is based, that practitioners will be helped to feel competent in the many areas of expanded practice in which they are often involved.

Although the book is primarily aimed at post registered nurses, nurses undergoing pre-registration nurse education will find this book helpful as they themselves will be involved to a limited extent in the practices described. The author welcomes comments and constructive criticism on this first edition.

M. Courtenay
January 2000

ACKNOWLEDGEMENTS

I would like to thank the staff at the Hillingdon Hospital Trust for their initial idea for the development of the distance learning packages that prompted the development of this book. I would also like to thank Paul Champion, Resuscitation Officer, South Buckinghamshire NHS Trust, Wycombe Hospital, for his advice and guidance. Finally, I would like to thank Michele Butler for her help in producing some of the anatomical and physiological knowledge presented in this text.

INTRODUCTION

Traditionally, healthcare professionals have had clearly defined roles. However, these traditional occupational boundaries have become blurred over recent years by the development of new roles. This is particularly evident in nursing, with the reduction in junior doctors' hours and the increased opportunities for nurses to expand their practice. Nurses are increasingly undertaking practices, e.g. venepuncture and intravenous cannulation, that were, until fairly recently, the exclusive province of doctors. Nurses are cast in such roles as nurse practitioners, clinical nurse specialists and advanced practitioners.

The Scope of Professional Practice[1] and *Code of Professional Conduct*[2] reflect the dynamic, responsive nature of nursing, midwifery and health-visiting practice and provide a clear framework for the logical development of advanced practitioner roles.[3] The personal responsibility and accountability of individual practitioners to protect and improve standards of care are emphasized in these documents. Within *The Scope of Professional Practice* the need for the individual to apply knowledge to practice and to exercise professional judgement and skills are underlined, the responsibility of the practitioner relating to their personal experience, education and skill. *The Scope of Professional Practice* highlights the need for nurses to acknowledge any limitations in their competence, and 'decline any duties unless they are able to perform them in a skilled manner'.

The expanded practices and new roles which nurses are currently under-taking are often in areas of specialism in which a sound knowledge of the life sciences is essential. Therefore, if practitioners are to expand as opposed to extend their roles, i.e. learn only discreet skills or tasks, an understanding of this knowledge is crucial.

This book examines a number of advanced nursing skills. The procedure for each skill is described and the research evidence upon which these procedures are based is provided. The knowledge from the life sciences that underpins these advanced nursing skills is also presented in each chapter. It is evident from the literature that many students studying the life sciences have anxieties. These anxieties focus on the relevance of the subjects to tasks performed,[4] the difficulties involved in understanding these sciences,[5] and the lack of appropriate knowledge to understand the physiological phenomena encountered in the clinical environment.[6] Therefore, the life science knowledge presented in this text is clearly linked to the advanced nursing skill described.

References

1. United Kingdom Central Council for Nursing, Midwifery, and Health Visiting *The Scope of Professional Practice* 1992; London: UKCC.

2. United Kingdom Central Council for Nursing, Midwifery, and Health Visiting *Code of Professional Conduct* 1992; London: UKCC.

3. Department of Health The extended role of the nurse/scope of professional practice [Letter from the CNO] 1992; London; DoH.

4. Akinsanya, J.A. The life sciences in nurse education. PhD thesis, 1982 University of London.

5. Courtenay, M. A study of the teaching and learning of the biological sciences in nurse education. *Journal of Advanced Nursing* 1991; 16: 1110–1116.

6. Leonard, A., Jowett, S. Charting the course: a study of the six ENB pilot schemes in pre-registration nurse education. Research paper no. 1. In *National Evaluation of Demonstration Schemes in Pre-registration Nurse Education* 1990; London: National Foundation for Educational Research in England and Wales.

VENEPUNCTURE

Venepuncture is the most commonly performed invasive procedure in the UK[1] and nursing staff are increasingly performing this practice. This chapter provides an initial overview of the vascular system and blood. This knowledge is then applied to the selection of appropriate sites upon which to perform venepunture and the techniques used to undertake this advanced nursing skill.

APPLIED ANATOMY AND PHYSIOLOGY

Vascular system

The vascular system refers to the system of blood vessels. Blood vessels form a network that transports blood away from the heart, carry it to body tissues and then return it to the heart. There are five main types of blood vessel:

- Arteries
- Arterioles
- Capillaries

- Venules
- Veins

Arteries

Arteries carry blood from the heart to the tissues. They have a hollow core or **lumen** through which blood flows and three coats. The inner coat of the arterial wall is the **tunica intima**; there is an endothelial lining in contact with the blood in the lumen; and a layer of elastic tissue. The **tunica media** or middle coat is composed of elastic fibres and smooth muscle and is the thickest layer. Finally the outer coat or **tunica adventitia** is composed mainly of elastic and collagen fibres (**Figure 1.1**).

Owing to the structure of the tunica media, arteries exhibit two major properties: elasticity and contractility. When the contracting ventricles of the heart eject blood into the large arteries, these arteries expand to accommodate for extra blood. Then during ventricular relaxation, elastic recoil of the arteries moves blood onwards. Smooth muscle arranged longitudinally and circularly around the lumen is responsible for contractility. Sympathetic nervous system stimulation will contract smooth muscle and narrow the lumen of the vessel.

ARTERY

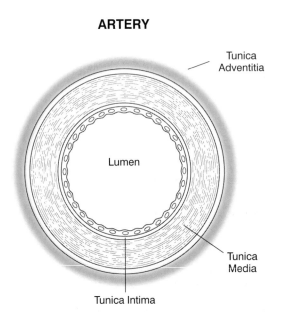

Figure 1.1 – Artery

This is called **vasoconstriction**. When sympathetic stimulation is removed, smooth muscle relaxes and the size of the lumen increases. This is known as **vasodilation**. Contractility also serves to control bleeding by causing vascular spasm. Blood flowing through an artery is under high pressure and large quantities of blood may be lost from a damaged artery.

Large arteries may be referred to as **conducting** or **elastic** arteries. Their tunica media contains more elastic tissue than smooth muscle, and these vessels conduct blood from the heart to the distribution system of arteries.

Medium-sized arteries may be referred to as distributing or muscular arteries. Their tunica media contains more smooth muscle than elastic tissue, and these vessels distribute blood to various body parts.

Medium-sized arteries will divide into small arteries, which in turn divide into much smaller vessels called **arterioles**.

Arterioles

These very small arteries are responsible for delivering blood to the capillaries. Arterioles close to the arteries from which they branch have a tunica media of smooth muscle with little elastic tissue. Arterioles closest to capillaries, however, consist of little more than an endothelial layer surrounded by a few smooth muscle cells. Arterioles offer considerable resistance to blood flow due to their small radius and are the main site of resistance to blood flow in the vascular system. During vasoconstriction in arterioles, blood flow into capillaries is restricted. When vasodilation occurs, blood flow into capillaries is drastically increased.

Capillaries

Capillaries, also known as **exchange vessels**, are microscopic vessels that connect arterioles and venules, and they are the part of the circulatory system where the exchange of gases, fluids, nutrients and metabolic wastes occurs between the blood and cells. They consist of a single layer of endothelium and a basement membrane. There is no tunica media or adventitia (**Figure 1.2**). Hence, substances present in the blood only have to pass through the cell membrane of just a single cell to reach tissue cells.

The distribution of capillaries throughout the body varies depending on how active a tissue is. Many capillaries are found in active tissues such as

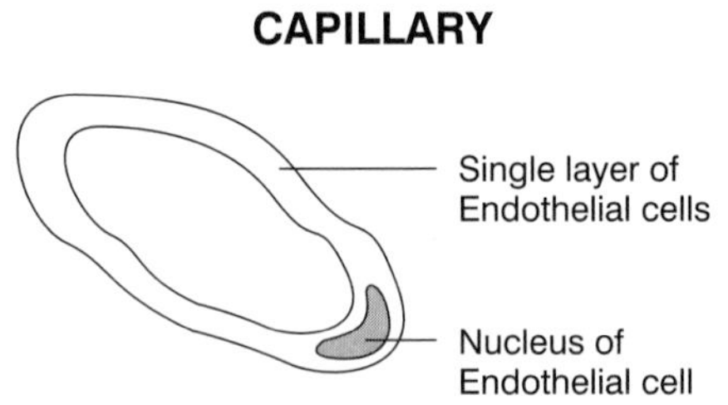

CAPILLARY

Single layer of
Endothelial cells

Nucleus of
Endothelial cell

Figure 1.2 – Capillary

muscle and liver, but are less common in tendons and ligaments. The cornea and epidermis are devoid of a capillary network.

When several capillaries merge they form small veins or **venules.**

Venules

Venules collect capillary blood and drain it into veins. Post-capillary venules are mainly of endothelium and a thin tunica adventitia. Venules approaching veins, however, possess a tunica media similar to veins (see below).

Veins

Veins return blood from the tissues back to the right side of the heart. The walls of veins consist of the same three layers as arteries. However, there is considerably less elastic tissue and smooth muscle tissue (**Figure 1.3**). The walls are thinner and more distensible and the diameter of the lumen is larger offering a lower resistance to blood flow. By the time that blood arrives in veins from capillaries and venules, it has lost a lot of pressure. This fall in pressure can be seen in the blood flow from a cut vein. Blood leaves the vein in an even flow rather than in high-pressure spurts characteristic of a cut artery.

Some veins, especially those in the arms and legs, have **valves.** Valves have two semilunar, internal folds of the tunica intima (endothelium) that permit blood to flow in only one direction, restricting any backflow. The presence of venous valves together with the skeletal muscle pump and the respiratory pump all assist venous return or return of blood to the heart.

The median cephalic and basilic veins in the antecubital fossa are normally used for taking blood, venepuncture. They are well supported by muscle and connective tissue, and are visible and easy to palpate.

VEIN

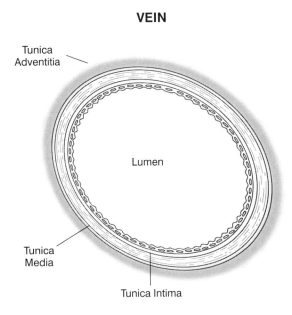

Figure 1.3 – Vein

BLOOD

Blood is circulated throughout the body by the pumping action of the heart and by the vascular system described above. Blood is required to perform the following functions:

- Transport of oxygen from the lungs to the tissues
- Transport of waste products of cell metabolism from tissues to the lungs, liver, kidneys and sweat glands
- Transport of nutrients, hormones, enzymes and other substances throughout the body
- Regulation of body temperature
- Regulation of acid–base balance, and water and electrolyte balance in body fluids
- Protection against microorganisms by contributing to the inflammatory and immune responses

The blood volume of an average adult is about 8% of total body weight. An average adult male has 5–6 litres of blood while an average adult female has 4–5 litres. Blood is thicker and denser than water due to the presence of erythrocytes (red blood cells) and plasma proteins. Blood specific gravity is between 1.045 and 1.065 and the pH ranges from 7.35 to 7.45, so making blood very slightly alkaline. Arterial blood appears red due to the haemoglobin being oxygenated, while venous blood (with oxygen removed) appears bluish or darker. Deoxygenated venous blood will, however, turn bright red as soon as it is exposed to oxygen in the air. This would be observed, for example, if a vein is cut.

Blood components

Blood consists of a liquid component called plasma and formed elements, which are mainly blood cells suspended in the plasma.

Plasma

Plasma is yellow and contains 90% water, which acts as the solvent for dissolving and transporting nutrients. The remaining 10% of plasma is composed of:

- Plasma proteins – globulins, albumins and fibrinogen
- Plasma electrolytes – include sodium, potassium, chloride, calcium, phosphate, iodide and magnesium
- Nutrients and waste products – include glucose, amino acids, lipids (triglycerides, free fatty acids, cholesterol, phospholipids), lactic acid, urea, creatinine
- Gases and buffers – include oxygen, carbon dioxide, nitrogen, bicarbonate
- Enzymes and hormones

Formed elements

These are mainly blood cells that can be subdivided into:

- *Erythrocytes* (red blood cells)

- *Leucocytes* (white blood cells) – these require further subdivision into:
  — Granulocytes
  — Neutrophils
  — Eosinophils
  — Basophils
- *Agranulocytes*
  — Lymphocytes (T- and B-cells)
  — Monocytes
- *Thrombocytes* (platelets)

Many of the blood components are routinely measured in clinical practice. The nurse will be required to undertake venepuncture to provide blood samples for common haematological or biochemical tests. The nurse should, therefore, be familiar with blood tests commonly undertaken and the requirements of each test. For example, the patient may need to be fasted before the test or a specific volume of blood may be required. Details of specific tests are beyond the scope of this book, however, and the reader should refer to Evans[2] or another relevant text for details of these and other blood tests for which they may be required to undertake. The haematology and biochemistry laboratories at local hospitals will also provide relevant information.

Selection of veins for venepuncture

There are factors that influence the choice of vein to use for venepuncture,[3] including:

- Age of the patient
- Previous uses and condition of the veins
- Patient's weight, i.e. obese or malnourished
- Clinical status of the patient, e.g. dehydrated, shock, amputee, oedema, thrombocytopaenic, stroke, mastectomy
- Other clinical procedures required during admission
- Type and length of treatment

- Medications, e.g. warfarin, steroids

- Patient preference (also ethnic and religious requirements)

- Patient cooperation/previous experiences

- If veins are required for chemotherapy

- If veins are impeded by fractures

Palpation of the veins prior to venepuncture enables the identification of a suitable vein. It also ensures that an artery is not mistaken for a vein. A vein can be emptied by digital pressure and is pulseless. It is also important during the assessment that any rashes or other dermatological conditions are identified. Patients likely to present with problems when performing venepuncture include: intravenous drug abusers, patients who have received extensive chemotherapy, and those with poor vascular circulation such as diabetics. The veins in these patients will often be hard and it may be very difficult to find an appropriate site. Similar problems may arise when performing venepuncture on the elderly as a result of poor circulation.

A good vein for venepuncture is:

- Bouncy

- Soft

- Refills when depressed

- Visible

- Has a large lumen

- Is well supported[3]

By contrast, veins to avoid, include those that are:

- Thrombosed/sclerosed/fibrosed (detected by a lack of resilience and a hard, cord like feeling)

- Inflamed/bruised

- Thin/fragile

- Mobile/tortuous

- Near bony prominences, painful

- Areas or sites of infection, oedema or phlebitis

- In the lower extremities, i.e. there is an increased risk of thrombophlebitis and pulmonary embolism

- Have undergone multiple punctures[3]

The superficial veins of the upper extremities of the body are located just beneath the skin (**Figure 1.4**) and are used for venepuncture.

The veins used for venepuncture are the median cephalic and basilic veins in the antecubital fossa. They are well supported by muscle and connective tissue, and are visible and easy to palpate. However, the median cephalic vein crosses in front of the brachial artery and care must be taken to avoid puncturing it.

Asepsis

Asepsis is vital to prevent contamination by microorganisms. Contamination can occur in two major ways:

- Direct contact from nurse to patient

- From the skin flora of the patient

To prevent the transmission of infection from practitioner to patient, effective handwashing and drying techniques are essential. Furthermore, as part of a universal precaution policy, gloves must be worn to protect the patient and practitioner from blood-borne infection.[4] To avoid the risk of contamination by the patient's skin flora, firm and prolonged rubbing (30 seconds to 1 minute) with an antiseptic solution such as chlorohexidine in

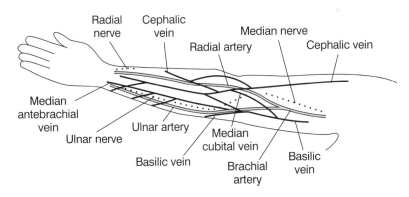

Figure 1.4(a) – The superficial blood vessels and nerves of the forearm

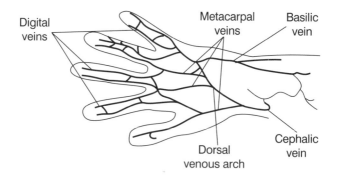

Figure 1.4(b) – The superficial veins of the hand

70% alcohol or 2% aqueous solution is recommended.[5] Once the skin has been cleaned and allowed to dry, the vein should not be touched or re-palpated. Any unwanted hair should be clipped with clean scissors as opposed to shaved.[3] Any abrasions which might be caused when shaving can harbour bacteria.[6,7]

Venous access

Methods of improving venous access include the application of a tourniquet to the upper arm. The tourniquet should not affect arterial flow but must be tight enough to impede venous return and to promote venous distension. Lightly tapping the vein will also cause the vein to distend and will improve access. However, if the vein is tapped too hard it can be painful and a haematoma may develop. This action could be considered an assault in a Court of Law. If each method fails, immersing the patients limb in warm water for several minutes or a warm compress should be tried.[3] As a last resort the patient could be asked to lower their hand below the level of their heart and make a fist. However, this can cause damage to the veins and should only be used if all other methods have been ineffective.

Venepuncture procedure

Once the insertion site has been cleaned, the needle guard should be removed and discarded. The bevelled edge of the needle should be positioned uppermost. The next step is to stabilize and anchor the vein with a hand or thumb below the insertion site. This immobilizes the vein and provides counter tension, which will facilitate the needle to move smoothly into the vein. The needle should be slid, as opposed to stabbed, into the selected vein and the blood withdrawn slowly ensuring haemolysis (rupture of red blood cells) does not occur. The tourniquet can then be released and the needle removed. The patient can be asked to press firmly on a clean piece of sterile gauze. If they cannot do this the tourniquet can be replaced over the gauze and used to apply gentle pressure until the site is dressed. Adhesive tape such as Elastoplast® (if the patient is not allergic to this material), or cottonwool and Micropore® should be applied once the site has stopped bleeding. If a suitable vein cannot be found, or if following two attempts there has been no success, help should be sought. Multiple unsuccessful attempts will limit future vascular access. Unnecessary trauma will also be caused to the patient. If during venepuncture bruising occurs, it is vital that the tourniquet is removed, as the vein wall may have been punctured.

After discarding the needle from the syringe into the sharps container, the blood can be distributed into the prepared and labelled bottles. The bottles containing anti-coagulants need to be mixed well and inverting the bottle will do this. Bottles for clotted specimens must be kept upright. This ensures that the clot forms uniformly in the bottom of the bottle as opposed to spreading along the sides. It is important to ensure that the containers are filled to the specified amount (particularly bottles for clotted specimens), because if they are not then laboratory equipment may be unable to read them or may give a false result necessitating further venepuncture.

Closed vacuum container systems

An alternative method for taking blood involves the use of closed vacuum container systems (**Figure 1.5**). In such a system the blood is collected via a needle directly into a specimen tube under a vacuum. Vacuum container systems are popular for reasons of safety, cost and convenience. When using these systems, screw the needle into the needle holder. Once again apply the tourniquet, palpate if necessary and select an appropriate vein. Clean the site to be used. The shield can then be removed from the needle and checked to ensure the bevel is uppermost. The next step is to stabilize and anchor the vein with a hand or thumb below the insertion site. Holding the complete unit between thumb and index finger, then penetrate the skin. When the needle is in place reverse the position of the hands. The collection tube can then be pressed with the thumb of the right hand (if right-handed); the index and the centre fingers supported on the flange of the holder. The vacuum enables the blood to flow, as the rubber seal of the tube passes over

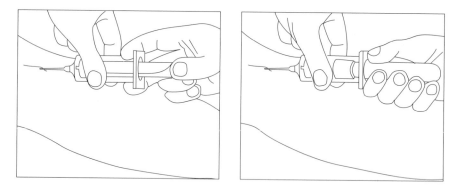

Figure 1.5 – Using a closed vacuum container system

the valved end of the needle. The tourniquet can be released as blood starts to flow. Following this procedure, the needle and holder can be withdrawn and the puncture site pressed firmly.

Health and safety issues

Needle-stick injuries from used needles are one of the greatest dangers to the practitioner while undertaking venepuncture. There is one needlestick injury for every 3000–4000 needle-handling procedures.[8] On removal of the needle, it must be placed in a sharps container. In an inoculation injury it is important that the wound is encouraged to bleed by firm squeezing and holding it under a tap of running warm water. The incident must be reported and officially documented, and advice sought from the occupational health department.

References

1. Peters, J.L., Frame, J.D., Dawson, S.M. Peripheral venous cannulation: reducing the risks. *British Journal of Parenteral Therapy* 1984; 5: 56–58.

2. Evans, D.M.D. *Special Tests* (14th edition), 1994; London: C.V. Mosby.

3. Dougherty, L. Intravenous cannulation. *Nursing Standard* 1996; 11(2): 47–54.

4. Schvarcz, R., Johansson, B., Nystrom, B., Sonnerborg, A. Nosocomial transmission of hepatitis C virus. *Infection* 1997; 25(2): 74–77.

5. Maki, D.G., Ringer, M., Alvarado, C.J. Prospective randomised trial of povadine iodine , alcohol, and chlorhexidine for prevention of infection associated with central venous and arterial catheters. *Lancet* 1991; 338: 339–343.

6. Terry, J., Baranowski, L., Lonsway, R.A., Hedick, C. *Intravenous Therapy: Clinical Principles and Practice* 1995; Philadelphia: W.B. Saunders.

7. Weinstein, S.M. *Plumer's Principles and Practice of Intravenous Therapy.* 1993; Philadelphia: J.B. Lippincott.

8. Goldwater, P.N., Law, R., Nixon, A.D. Impact of recapping device on venepuncture-related needlestick injury. *Infection Control and Hospital Epidemiology* 1989; 10(1): 21–25.

Review questions

1. Veins and arteries have the same types of tissues in their walls. However, these tissues are in different proportions. Draw and label a diagram showing a cross-section of both an artery and a vein.

2. How does the structure of an artery change during its progression from a major artery to an arteriole?

3. What are the three mechanisms that assist in venous return?

4. Identify three veins in the arm that may be used for venepuncture.

5. A 42-year-old man is malnourished and has been admitted for blood tests. He has had several recent and unsuccessful experiences of venepuncture in the antecubital fossa, which is now bruised and painful.

   • The patient is extremely anxious. Will this affect his veins? How?

   • What interventions might you employ to improve venous access?

   • Which veins would you avoid using?

6. Why are the median cubital veins impractical for venepuncture?

7. Consider a patient undergoing venepuncture. What steps should be taken throughout the procedure to prevent the development of infection in both the patient and practitioner?

8. What special precautions are necessary when taking blood from a patient with delayed clotting times?

9. What needle gauge should be used for venepuncture, and why?

10. Describe the advantages and disadvantages of a closed vacuum container system.

Review questions – answers

1. See pages 2–4

2. As arteries branch in their progress through the body, they become smaller with regards to diameter. Furthermore, the proportion of elastic tissue becomes less. The proportion of smooth muscle in the artery wall increases. This muscle enables the lumen of the artery to be increased and decreased, i.e. vasodilation and vasoconstriction.

3. Venous valves, skeletal muscle pump, respiratory pump.

4. Basilic vein, median cephalic vein, cephalic vein.

5.
   - Fear of the procedure could trigger a response of the autonomic nervous system. This is known as a vasovagal reaction and could cause syncope and vasoconstriction and subsequent limited venous access.

   - Application of a tourniquet, stroking of the vein, warm compresses or immersion of the limb in warm water.

   - Veins that relate to the bruised area for fear of causing further inflammation/extravasation

6. They cross an artery

7. Wear gloves when dealing with all risk patients and when performing blood culture procedures, effective hand washing and effective cleaning of the patient's skin, correct disposal of all equipment.

8. Ensure that they have stopped bleeding.

9. 22G. 21G should be used if there is a need for rapid blood flow.

10.
   - Advantages – closed vacuum container systems are leak-proof and airtight (closed system). Blood collection is faster and is safer with regards to spillage and contamination. There is decreased trauma to the veins, and only the required amount of blood is drawn. The risk of haemolysis is reduced. The container is used within the laboratory.

   - Disadvantages – unless the practitioner is experienced with the system there is a greater chance of causing trauma. There is no appearance of 'flashing' of blood into the needle hub. Difficult veins may sometimes be more of a problem, and a butterfly needle in conjunction with the system may be necessary.

2

PERIPHERAL INTRAVENOUS CANNULATION

Nurses involved in caring for patients with an IV cannula are increasingly taking over the process of cannulation.[1] A description of the vascular system and blood was presented in **Chapter 1**. Here, this knowledge is applied to the selection of appropriate sites on which to perform IV cannulation. This is followed by an examination of the IV cannulation procedure, including the preparation of the patient, selection of cannula and health and safety issues.

Selection of veins for intravenous cannulation

The factors that influence the choice of vein for IV cannulation, the characteristics of a good vein on which to perform this technique and patients likely to experience problems when undergoing this procedure are the same as in venepuncture and as described in **Chapter 1**.

As in venepuncture, the superficial veins of the upper extremities of the body are used for IV cannulation (**Figure 1.4**). Experienced practitioners should only use ankle and foot veins if there are no other suitable veins. However, patients suffering from diabetes should never be cannulated in these areas. The following factors need to be considered before cannulating these vessels:

- Digital veins should only be used as a last resort as they can only accommodate a very small gauge needle.

- Metacarpal veins, formed by the unison of digital veins, are easily visualized and palpable and so are more accessible and are a very good choice. However, in the elderly, where skin turgor and subcutaneous tissue is diminished, these veins are contraindicated.

- The cephalic vein due to its position and size makes it a very good choice for IV cannulation. However, complications such as mechanical phlebitis may be increased due to its position at a joint.

- The basilic vein, although more difficult to access as a result of its position, and the presence of valves, is frequently overlooked for the purpose of IV cannulation. However, valves can interfere with the advancement of cannulae.[2]

The site selected for IV cannulation should be on the distal part of the patient's limb, but proximal to previous attempts.[3] Cannulae inserted distally to previous attempts may cause irritant substances to pass an area of inflammation, which may prolong the inflammatory response. Also, leakage from the initial puncture site may cause an extravasation injury.

Asepsis

Almost 4000 cases of line-associated bacteraemia were reported in England and Wales in 1991.[4] *Staphylococcus aureus* and *Staphylococcus epidermis* are the most commonly responsible organisms.[5,6] Major infective complications documented in the literature include septic shock, sustained sepsis, suppurative thrombophlebitis, endocarditis, metastatic infection and arteritis.[7] Therefore, asepsis is vital to prevent contamination by microorganisms. The procedure for asepis during IV cannulation is as for venepuncture (see **Chapter 1**).

Preparation of the patient for peripheral intravenous cannulation

Before IV cannulation it is essential to ensure that the patient has a clear understanding of what the procedure involves, and that informal verbal consent is obtained. Furthermore, by ensuring that the patient is relaxed and their anxieties alleviated, vasoconstriction, one of the body's responses to stress, is prevented. The need for analgesia before IV cannulation should be decided on an individual basis. Topical creams or gels, such as Ametop® or Emla®, or intradermal injection of lignocaine, can be used for local anaesthesia. Lignocaine, e.g. Emla® a topical anaesthetic, can prove effective, although it must be applied 1 hour before cannulation, and it can cause vasoconstriction.[8] Local anaesthesia should not be used if pain, associated with the extravasation of vesicant solutions, is obscured. Good technique and vein selection are the most crucial factors influencing the pain experienced by the patient during cannulation.[2]

Selection of cannula

Following an assessment of the condition and accessibility of the patient's veins, the cannula can be selected. Just as there are patients with different disease complications and problems, there are different cannulae to suit each individual. Many of the newer cannulae are thin walled so that a large internal diameter is provided. However, the diameters of these devices vary, with a variety of gauges from 12 to 26. Precision engineering of the bevelled steel needle means that most cannula are V-shaped, so that the point of the needle gives a sharper, smoother insertion. There are certain catheters that, when inserted, are warmed by the body and softened to comply with the vessel within which they lie. These catheters reduce kinking and trauma on insertion and so reduce the risk of phlebitis.

General guidance governing the choice of cannulae recommends that the smallest possible gauge of cannula that suits the present or recognized future needs of the device should be used, and that this should be positioned in the largest vein possible.[9] This allows for the efficient haemodilution of substances as they are administered intravenously, and reduces the incidence of chemical infusion phlebitis. Cannulae also have to be selected with regard to the choice of material from which they are made. Polyurethane is less phlebitic than other materials and is softer, reducing the problem of mechanical damage.[10,11] Some general guidance on cannula selection is given in **Table 2.1**.

Table 2.1 – Guidelines for cannula selection[12]

Cannula size	Cannula situation
Gauge 14–16	Large volumes of fluid replacement e.g. major surgery
Gauge 18	Fast transfusion e.g. routine blood transfusions
Gauge 20	Bolus drug administration or routine transfusion
Gauge 22	Fragile and small veins. Only use for short-term access
Gauge 24	Fragile and small veins

INTRAVENOUS CANNULATION PROCEDURE

As for venepuncture (see **Chapter 1**) several methods can be applied to improve venous access. Following the cleaning of the insertion site, the vein must not be re-palpated or the skin touched. The vein should then be anchored and stabilized with a hand or thumb below the point of insertion. The vein is immobilized and counter tension provided. This enables the needle to move smoothly into the vein. To ensure that the cannula is inserted correctly it should be held by the flash chamber with the bevel of the needle in an upright position. To minimize damage to non-venous tissue, insertion should take place immediately over the chosen peripheral vein, at an angle of between 10° and 45° according to the depth of the vein in the subcutaneous tissue.[2] By placing the cannula in line with the vein, manipulation of the device under the skin is avoided and tissue damage and bleeding prevented. Successful entry is indicated by flashback of blood into the chamber of the stylet.[2]

After the cannula has been inserted, decreasing the cannula angle slightly should level the device, and the cannula can be slowly advanced to ensure entry into the lumen of the vein. The stylet can next be withdrawn slightly and a second flashback of blood should be seen along the shaft of the cannula.[2] The cannula can then be advanced into the vein, anchoring the vein at the same time. At this point the tourniquet can be released, pressure applied to the vein above the cannula and the stylet removed. The cannula should be secured in position following the attachment of a giving set or other appropriate device. A poorly secured catheter will cause discomfort for the patient and will increase the risk of thrombophlebitis with the associated complications of infection and pain. Clean tape can be used for this procedure as long as it is applied over the top of an IV dressing product. The tape should not come into contact with the insertion site nor obscure it. The site must be inspected regularly for signs of phlebitis, infiltration, leakage, infection and bleeding. The main aim of cannula site management is to prevent the accumulation of moisture. Occlusive dressings are associated with the accumulation of moisture (under the dressing) and microbial growth.[4] It is essential that IV products, e.g. Opsite®, IV 3000®, and Vecafix®, are used to dress infusion devices as opposed to wound-care products. Dry sterile gauze is also an effective dressing as it maintains dryness at the entry site. Bandaging is not necessary and should be avoided as it obscures visual assessment.

If, on the first attempt, cannulation is unsuccessful, the stylet should never be re-inserted. This could result in a catheter embolism. The cut part of the catheter may be carried away in the venous return to the heart. This could then become a focus for infection, possibly lodged in the pulmonary arterial system. 'Multiple septic complications' as a cause of mortality secondary to IV cannulation have also been reported.[13] A second attempt at cannulation should be proximal to the first. If this proves unsuccessful, an experienced nurse or physician should evaluate the patient's venous access. Only if venous access is adequate should further attempts be made.[3] Future vascular access will be limited by multiple unsuccessful attempts and the patient will suffer undue trauma. As in venepuncture, the tourniquet should be removed if there is bruising during the procedure as the wall of the vein may have been punctured. The haematoma will be reduced by the application of pressure and a cold pack to the vessel.

Following siting of the cannula, it should be flushed with 5–10 ml normal saline. This technique ensures the patency of the device.

The following details should also be documented:

- Patient's name and hospital number.
- Name of the person who undertook the cannulation procedure (both printed and signed).
- Date and time.
- Site of access.
- Device and methods used.
- Reason for cannulation.
- Number of attempts.
- Any problems or complications encountered and how they were dealt with.

It is essential that the cannulation site is inspected during each nursing shift for signs of phlebitis or infiltration. Although it may be difficult to achieve in certain groups of patients, it is it is recommended[14] that to reduce the risk of phlebitis, peripheral cannula should be re-sited every 48–72 hours. During the removal of cannula, care must be taken not to damage the vein. Pressure must also be applied for 1 minute to stop the bleeding. A sterile dressing should then cover the site.

HEALTH AND SAFETY ISSUES

As in venepuncture, one of the greatest dangers to the practitioner while undertaking peripheral IV cannulation is needle-stick injuries from used needles. Once the needle is removed from the cannula, it must be placed in a sharps container. An innoculation injury should be dealt with as for venepuncture.

Protective devices have been developed to protect the user from blood spillages when there is a risk of infection, e.g. in the hepatitis and HIV patient. These cannula are made from Teflon and have a side arm that offers a remote injection facility. This reduces the risk of cannula movement and thereby protects against blood flush-back. However, unless cannulating in the trauma setting, one is unlikely to come into contact with blood if cannulating proficiently.

Other protective devices include retractable cannula needles. Manufacturers have now developed an apparatus in which the needle is withdrawn from the cannula on insertion. The needle is enclosed within a protective case preventing further contact. These devices are commonly used in the USA. However, they are also beginning to be used in the UK by paramedics, known HIV and AIDS patients, and accident departments. Unfortunately, these devices are more expensive than the standard cannula and it prohibits their general use.

References

1. Peters, J.L., Frame, J.D., Dawson, S.M. Peripheral venous cannulation: reducing the risks. *British Journal of Parenteral Therapy* 1984; 5: 56–58.

2. Dougherty, L. Intravenous cannulation. *Nursing Standard* 1996; 11(2): 47–54

3. Terry, J., Baranowski, L., Lonsway, R.A., Hedick, C. *Intravenous Therapy: Clinical Principles and Practice.* 1995; Philadelphia: W.B. Saunders.

4. Elliot, T.S.J. Line associated bacteraemias. *Communicable Disease Report* 1993; 3(7): R91–96

5. Elliot, T.S., Faroqui, M.H. Infections and intravascular devices. *British Journal of Hospital Medicine* 1992; 48(8): 496–503

6. Fry, D.E., Fry, R.V., Borzotta, A. P. Nosocomial blood borne infection secondary to intravascular devices. *American Journal of Surgery* 1994; 167(2): 268–272.

7. Arnow, P.M., Quimosing, E.M., Beach, M. Consequences of intravascular catheter sepsis. *Clinical Infectious Diseases* 1993; 16(6): 778–784.

8. Gunwardene, R.D., Davenport, H.T. Local applications of Emla and Glycryl Trinitrate ointment before venepuncture. *Anaesthesia* 1990; 45: 52–54

9. Angles, T., Barbone, M. Infiltration and phlebitis: assessment, management and documentation. *Journal of Home Health Care Practice* 1994; 7(1): 16–21

10. Gaukroger, P.B., Roberts, J.G., Maners, T.A. Infusion thrombophlebitis: a prospective comparison of 645 Vialon and Teflon cannulae in anaesthetic and postoperative use. *Anaesthesia and Intensive Care* 1988; 16(3): 265–271.

11. Stonehouse, J., Butcher, J. Phlebitis associated with peripheral cannulae. *Professional Nurse* 1996; 12(1): 51–54.

12. Jackson, A. Performing peripheral intravenous cannulation. *Professional Nurse* 1997; 13(1): 21–25.

13. Frieberg, D.M., Barnes, D.J. Fatal sepsis following peripheral intravenous cannula embolus. *Chest* 1992; 101(3): 865–866.

14. Goodison, S.M. Good practice ensures minimum risk factors. *Professional Nurse* 1990; 6(3): 175–177.

Review questions

1. You are asked to cannulate an 82-year-old man who is receiving anticoagulant therapy. What problems might you may encounter and how could you alleviate or prevent them?

2. Identify the median cubital veins on your own arm. Why are they impractical for cannulation?

3. A 26-year-old man is admitted for antibiotic therapy. Although never cannulated before, he has had several recent and unsuccessful experiences of venepuncture in the antecubital fossa, which is now bruised and painful.

   - The patient is anxious about the procedure. How will this effect his veins?

   - Which veins would you avoid using and why?

   - What complications may arise as a result of his drug therapy?

4. Consider a patient with an IV infusion. Identify the possible portals of entry, from the cannula insertion site to the fluid insertion container, whereby bacteria may enter the system. How can this risk be minimized?

5. How could anxiety affect a patient's veins?

6. What factors would you consider when selecting a cannula?

7. What should you not do once you have cleaned the skin in preparation for cannulation?

8. Imagine that a thin, frail, elderly patient with weak thin-walled veins requires IV fluids 4 hourly. What gauge would you consider the most suitable and why?

9. Having a cannula inserted is painful. What measures can be taken to minimize the pain, and which cannulae are more easily inserted in view of their design?

Review questions – answers

1.
- Risk of bruising if a tourniquet is used
- Bleeding if the patient or practitioner does not apply pressure for 5 min
- Previous bruises/haematoma from venepuncture/cannulation which restricts sites

2. They cross an artery

3.
- Fear of the procedure could trigger a response of the autonomic nervous system. This is known as a vasovagal reaction and could cause syncope and vasoconstriction and subsequent limited venous access
- Veins that relate to the bruised area may cause further inflammation/ extravasation depending on infusate through the cannula
- Delayed inflammatory response; extravasation depending on the drug; chemical phlebitis and increased pressure on the vein if administered to quickly

4. Possible portals of entry
- Insertion site
- Ports e.g. three-way tap
- Injection site
- Connection sites
- Fluid contaminants
- Contaminated skin flora

Prevention
- Correct gauge, cannula, vein
- Ensure equipment is sterile
- Cleanse skin
- Non-use of ported systems if they can be avoided
- Observe site regularly

5. Fear of the procedure could trigger a response of the autonomic nervous system. This is known as a vasovagal reaction and could cause syncope and vasoconstriction and subsequent limited venous access

6.
- What the cannula will be used for, e.g. blood, bolus injection
- Type of vein/condition of patient
- Whether a 'longer stay' cannula, e.g. Optiva®, is required
- Flow rate required
- Selection of a cannula for a secure fix

7. Palpate the area once more

8. 22 or 24G Optiva® as this expands and the lumen has a larger diameter

9. V-shaped cannula precision bevelled, e.g. Optiva® and Optiva® 2. Local anaesthesia, e.g. Ametop gel, as this vasodilates and anaesthetizes within 30 minutes

INTRAVENOUS DRUG ADMINISTRATION

The shift in responsibility for the delivery of intravenous (IV) therapy from doctors to nurses began around the time of the Second World War. Staff shortages and the acceptance by nurses to extend their practice drove this development. Today, *The Scope of Professional Practice*,[1] in conjunction with the reduction in junior doctors' hours, has allowed nurses to establish a niche in the area of IV fluid and drug delivery. It is now common practice in the majority of clinical settings for nurses to be responsible for this advanced nursing skill. An overview of the vascular system and blood was presented in **Chapter 1**. Here, this knowledge is applied to the methods by which IV drugs are administered, and the advantages and disadvantages of this route are highlighted. The major hazards associated with IV therapy and infection control issues are then examined. Finally, the types of infusion devices used for IV fluid and drug delivery are described.

METHODS OF INTRAVENOUS DRUG ADMINISTRATION

The methods by which nurses are able to administer IV drugs include:

- Continuous infusion

- Intermittent infusion

- Direct intermittent injection

Continuous infusion

Continuous infusion involves the administration of a volume of fluid over a number of hours, and the task may be repeated over days. The method is used when the drug needs to be highly diluted and the maintenance of steady blood drug levels is necessary.[2] This method usually always involves infusion control devices to regulate the rate of infusion delivery, ensuring that the correct rate and volume of drug is given. During the administration of a continuous infusion, it is important that where possible pre-prepared infusion fluids with additives are used. If additions are necessary, it is essential to ensure that these additions are compatible. Multiple drug additions should be avoided, and only one addition should be added to the fluid bag. Additions must not be added to total parenteral nutrition (TPN) because TPN provides an ideal medium for bacterial growth and will also precipitate out in the presence of electrolytes and drugs. The only additions that should be made to TPN are vitamins, which must be authorized by a pharmacist. TPN should always be administered through a dedicated feeding line. The use of three-way taps should be avoided because they act as a reservoir for microorganisms.[3]

Following the addition of a drug to infusion fluids, the solution must be mixed well to prevent a layering effect, which can happen with some drugs. e.g. potassium chloride (KCl). Additions should, therefore, be made before the infusion fluid being hung on the infusion stand. The fluid bag should be labelled clearly following the addition,[2] and the patient and the infusion fluid monitored closely during administration.

Intermittent infusion

This method involves the infusion of a small volume i.e. 50–250 ml, during an interval of 20 minutes to 2 hours. An intermittent infusion may be given as one specified dose or at a number of intervals over 24 hours. This type of infusion is administered when:

- The drug pharmacology requires this dilution.

- A large volume infusion would render the drug unstable.

- Large volumes of fluid are not appropriate for the patient.

- The patient requires a peak plasma level.[2]

A 'Y set' or a burette set with a 100 or 150 ml chamber capacity may be used to deliver a drug by intermittent infusion. If fluids are not needed between doses, a small volume infusion can be connected to a heparinized cannula.[2] As in a continuous infusion, pre-prepared infusion fluids with additives should be used. Multiple drug additions should be avoided. Following the addition of a drug to infusion fluids, the solution must be mixed well and clearly labelled. During administration, the patient and the infusion fluid should be closely monitored.

Direct intermittent injection

This method requires that the injection of a small volume of drug is given via a cannula, through a re-sealable bung, extension set or the injection site of an administration set, over several seconds or minutes using a syringe and needle.[2] Whatever the method selected it is essential that the practitioner, before administering the drug, removes any bandages and examines the cannula insertion site and ensures the patency of the vein.

This form of injection may be used in the following situations:[2]

- A bolus injection in an emergency, given rapidly over a few seconds when a maximum concentration of the drug is required by vital organs.

- If, due to pharmacological or therapeutic reasons, the drug cannot be diluted. The drug is given as a controlled injection over a few minutes.

- When a peak blood level is required and this is unable to be achieved by a small volume infusion.

Drug compatability must be ensured if drugs are administered into an infusion injection site. Normal saline can be used to flush the line if the infusion fluid is incompatible with the drug to be administered.[2] A weak solution of heparin can be used to maintain cannula patency.

Reheparinisation should occur regularly to prevent the formation of fibrin. Reheparinisation is necessary following the administration of each drug.[2] Normal saline must be used between each drug and at the end of drug administration if multiple drugs are administered.[2] The patient must be observed for any pain or discomfort, swelling or redness at the insertion site. Detection of extravasation is essential.

ADVANTAGES OF INTRAVENOUS DRUG ADMINISTRATION

Advantages of the IV route for drug administration include:[4]

- The rapid rise in plasma levels of the drug enables dosage to be titrated with the desired effect. This ensures that the minimum therapeutic dose is given, preventing any possible side-effects.

- Rapid action of the drug.

- The total absorption of the drug enables the precise dose of the drug to be calculated, thus making the treatment more reliable.

- The volume of fluid injected IV allows potentially irritating preparations to be diluted. Furthermore, any pain or irritation that may be caused by substances given subcutaneously or intramuscularly is avoided.

- The therapeutic effect can be modified or maintained due to the rate of administration being controlled.

- Drugs that cannot be absorbed by any other route can be given.

- Once a cannula has been inserted and secured, injections are painless.

DISADVANTAGES OF INTRAVENOUS DRUG ADMINISTRATION

Disadvantages of the IV route for drug administration include:[4]

- The action of the drug is rapid. Unwanted effects are also rapid and it is impossible to stop the action of the drug.

- Fluid and drug incompatibility may cause precipitate formation and the formation of new compounds.

- Allergy and anaphylaxis to an injected drug.

- The accumulation of toxic concentrations of the drug in the plasma as a result of the drug being given too rapidly can result in 'speed shock'. Symptoms include a flushed face, headache, congestion and tightness in the chest, and an irregular pulse. Tachycardia, acute hypotension, syncope and cardiac arrest are more dangerous symptoms.

- Extravasation – this is the infusion of drugs or fluid into the tissues instead of the venous circulation. Fluids that are alkaline or acidic, cytotoxic, vasoconstricting or hypertonic may be irritating to tissue and lead to necrosis. These are called vesicant fluids and must be monitored closely. In the event of extravasation the infusion must be stopped and medical advice sought.

- Particulate contamination, i.e. the injection of packaging debris – including rubber and glass – that are drawn up with the drug. This has been linked with lesions in the lungs, kidney, spleen, liver and brain. The use of small-gauge needles for aspiration, filter needles and in-line filters helps prevent it.

The problems associated with intravenous therapy

IV fluids and drugs may be administered either centrally or peripherally. Peripheral lines carry less risk than central lines. The problems associated with peripheral cannulae include:[4]

- Infiltration

- Extravasation

- Phlebitis

- Haematoma

The problems associated with central lines are predominantly associated with the cannulation process or management of the IV therapy and include:

- Air embolism

- Pneumothorax

- Haemorrhage

- Local nerve injury

- Arterial puncture

- Thromboembolism

- Infection (local or systemic)

- Tamponade

- Dyssrhythmias

- Catheter embolism[3]

Problems such as drug toxicity, fluid overload, anaphylaxis and speed shock are complications that can be common to both the peripheral and central routes of access.

The major hazards associated with intravenous therapy

The major hazards associated with IV therapy are thrombophlebitis, bacteraemia and septicaemia.[5]

Thrombophlebitis

Thrombophlebitis is the inflammation of a vein and is associated with thrombus formation. The condition can cause infiltration, oedema, haemorrhage and necrosis of the vein wall.[5]

Bacteraemia

When there is no other primary focus for infection and there is microbiological evidence of intravascular cannula infection, cannula-related sepsis is defined as bacteraemia or fungaemia.[5] Vascular catheter-related infection is an important cause of mortality and morbidity in the hospitalized patient (see **Chapter 2**)

Suppurative thrombophlebitis

This condition occurs most commonly when plastic catheters have been left *in situ* for longer than 48–72 hours[5] and involves a lethal infection of a vein segment. In some cases purulent drainage can be seen at the cannula site.

Some causative factors have been linked with thrombophlebitis and sepsis:

- Chemical factors involving the infusate
- Cannula composition
- Dressings
- Disinfectant
- Asepsis in site preparation[5]

Thrombophlebitis may start as a localized response to chemical or physical irritation. However, it can rapidly develop into bacteraemia or suppurative thrombophlebitis. The foreign material of the cannula activates the blood clotting mechanism causing thrombus development. Thrombi then become a focus for bacterial proliferation. The skin flora of patients or staff, contaminated equipment, and other sites of infection such as wounds, can all be sources of microorganisms. Fragmentation of thrombi will cause the infection to spread.

Infection control

Aseptic technique must be followed throughout all IV procedures (see **Chapter 1**). This includes effective handwashing and drying techniques. Before the administration of IV drugs, an alcohol-based antiseptic solution should be used to clean injection sites or bungs.[3] They should be allowed to dry. It is desirable to have as few connections or stopcocks as possible in the IV infusion system to reduce the risk of contamination. Three-way taps act as a reservoir for microorganisms[2] and should be avoided where possible. If such a tap is used it must be cleaned with a 70% alcohol solution before access and remain covered when not in use.[6]

Although the incidence of IV fluid contamination is rare, 24 hours is the maximum period that an IV fluid container should remain in use.[2] Blood transfusions should not be used for more than 4 hours[7] and lipid emulsions no longer than 12 hours.[8] IV giving-sets should be changed every 72 hours with the exception of TPN, which should be changed every 24 hours.[9–11]

The procedure for IV cannulation is described in **Chapter 2**. When re-dressing an IV site, an aseptic technique should be used and a sterile dressing applied. The dressing type and condition of the patient will determine the frequency of dressing change. If a gauze dressing has been used it will need to be changed every time the site is inspected. This will normally be at each drug administration or if the site is wet. If the dressing is transparent it can be left on peripheral cannula for the duration of cannula insertion.[12] However, this is provided that the cannula is replaced every 48–72 hours. The time that a dressing can be safely left on a central venous catheter has not yet been identified.[13] The time will depend on the condition of the patient and the cannulation site.

A non-touch technique should be used when dealing with bottles and infusion bags. Fluid must be observed for contamination, i.e. cloudiness or discoloration or the presence of particles. The cannula should be removed if there is any redness, swelling or if the patient is pyrexic. The patient should then be investigated for infection.

Table 3.1 highlights the areas of responsibility of the nurse administering IV drugs.

Table 3.1 *– Areas of responsibility of the nurse administering IV drug[3]*

- Ensuring the administration of the correct drug to the correct patient
- Drug compatibility with infusate
- Confirming patient electrolyte and drug levels if necessary
- Reconstitution of the drug
- Examination and assessment of the cannula site
- Maintenance of asepsis when administering drugs
- Flushing of cannula between drug doses
- Monitoring rate of drug administration
- Monitoring the patient
- Accurate record-keeping

INFUSION DEVICES

Gravity-controlled devices

Although there is a general trend away from gravity-controlled devices towards volumetric pumps and syringe drivers, intermittent and continuous infusions are still frequently regulated using this method.[14] Gravity-driven devices use gravity as the infusion method and, therefore, deliver fluid at a very low pressure. Drip rate controllers, used to monitor flow rate, are suitable for use with non-viscous IV infusions, i.e. IV fluids and blood products.

Electronic pumps

Syringe pumps are electronic pumps that deliver fluid under positive pressure. The pumps have a range of features and alarms. Syringe sizes usually range from 5 to 60 ml. This type of device can deliver infusions accurately at low flow rates (rates range from 0.5 to 200 ml/hour). Syringe pumps are usually used to deliver IV drugs and can be used for intermittent or continuous infusions. Syringe drivers are usually smaller but work in the same way as syringe pumps. These devices are usually used for the administration of subcutaneous infusions. Volumetric pumps, also an electronic pump, deliver a specific volume of fluid over a set period. They normally have alarms and a display screen. These pumps can deliver large volumes of fluid at low flow rates. The flow rate is calculated by volume and can range from 1.0 to 999 ml/hour in the adult. Micro-pumps are available for children and have smaller flow rates. Volumetric pumps can be used to deliver continuous or intermittent infusion.

Mechanical pumps

Mechanical pumps are useful in ambulatory use. They are not heavy and do not require an external power source. Elastometric pumps are mechanical and are employed in the IV administration of drugs such as antibiotics and cytotoxics.

References

1. United Kingdom Central Council for Nursing, Midwifery, and Health Visiting *The Scope of Professional Practice* 1992; London: UKCC.

2. Mallet, J., Bailey, C. *The Royal Marsden NHS Trust Manual of Clinical Nursing Procedures* (4th Edition). 1996; Oxford: Blackwell Science.

3. Scales, K. Practical and professional aspects of IV therapy. *Professional Nurse* 1997 (Supplement); 12: 8, s3–s5.

4. Campbell, J. Intravenous therapy. *Professional Nurse* 1996; 11: 7, 437–442.

5. Goodison, S.M. The risks of IV therapy. *Professional Nurse* 1990; February: 235–238.

6. Brosnan, K.M., Parham, A.M., Rutledge, B. *et al.* Stopcock contamination. *American Journal of Nursing* 1988; 88: 30, 320–324.

7. McClelland, B. (ed.) *Transfusion Medicine Handbook: Blood Transfusion Service of the United Kingdom* (2nd edition). 1996; London: DoH.

8. Jarvis, W.R., Highsmith, A.K., Allen, J.R., Haley, R.W. Bacterial growth and endo-toxin production in lipid emulsion. *Journal of Clinical Microbiology* 1984; 19: 17–20.

9. Snydman, D.R., Donnelly-Reidy, M., Perry, L.K., Martin, W.J. Intravenous tubing burettes can be safely changed at 72-hour intervals. *Infection Control* 1987; 8: 113–116.

10. Josephson, A., Gombert, M.E., Sierra, M.F. *et al.* The relationship between intravenous fluid contamination and the frequency of tubing replacement. *Infection Control* 1985; 6: 367–370.

11. Maki, D.G., Botticelli, J.T., LeRoy, M.L., Thielke, T.S. Prospective study of replacing administration sets for intravenous therapy at 48 vs 72 hour intervals. 72 hours is safe and cost effective. *Journal of the American Medical Association* 1987; 258: 1777–1781.

12. Maki, D.G., Ringer, M. Evaluation of dressing regimens for prevention of infection with peripheral intravenous catheters: gauze, a transparent polyurethane dressing and an iodophor transparent dressing. *Journal of the American Medical Association* 1987; 258: 2396–2403.

13. Pearson, M.L. Hospital infection practices advisory committee. Guidelines for prevention of intravascular device-related infections. *Infection Control and Hospital Epidemiology* 1996; 17: 438–473.

14. Woollons, S. Selection of intravenous infusion pumps. *Professional Nurse* (Supplement); 12(8): S14–S15.

Review questions

1. Consider a patient with a closed IV system from the cannula insertion site to the fluid insertion container. Identify the possible sites whereby bacteria may enter the system.

2. How can this risk be minimized?

3. Identify three advantages of IV drug administration (see page 6)

4. Identify three disadvantages of IV drug administration (see page 7)

5. What are the major hazards associated with IV therapy?

6. What is the maximum period that an IV container should remain in use?

7. With the exception of TPN, how frequently should IV giving-sets be changed?

Review questions – answers

1. Possible sites

   - Insertion site
   - Ports, e.g. three-way tap
   - Injection site
   - Connection sites
   - Fluid contaminants
   - Usage
   - Contaminated skin flora

2. *Prevention*

   - Correct gauge, cannula, vein
   - Ensure equipment is sterile
   - Cleanse skin
   - The non use of ported systems, if they can be avoided
   - Observe site regularly
   - Clear instructions to patient
   - Speedy removal of cannula if signs of infection appear

3. *See page 6*

4. *See page 7*

5. *Thrombophlebitis*

   - Bacteraemia
   - Septicaemia

6. *24 hours*

7. *Every 72 hours*

4

READING AND INTERPRETING THE ELECTROCARDIOGRAM

Electrodes placed on the body's surface can detect electrical activity, which occurs in the heart. The recording of these electrical events comprises an electrocardiogram. Comparison of the information obtained from electrodes, placed in different positions on the body, enables electrical activity to be monitored and so the performance of different areas of cardiac tissue. This chapter commences with a review of the cardiovascular system and electrophysiology. This is followed by an examination of the conduction system of the heart and the electrocardiogram. The identification of normal and abnormal heart rhythms is then described.

APPLIED ANATOMY AND PHYSIOLOGY

Circulatory system

Blood flows through the body in a closed network called the circulatory system. It is pumped from the left atrium of the heart into the left ventricle, ejected into the aorta and then into other arteries. Arteries carry the blood away from the heart. Each artery branches about 15–20 times, becoming smaller and smaller. These small arteries, or arterioles, which lead into a network of minute capillaries. Oxygen and nutrients diffuse through the thin walls of these vessels into the tissues of the body. The capillaries eventually form venules, which lead onto veins. Veins take the blood back to the right side of the heart, entering the right atrium via the vena cavae. The right ventricle then pumps this blood to the lungs where it becomes oxygenated, and then it returns to the left side of the heart.

The heart, like other organs, also requires an adequate supply of oxygen and nutrients. These are supplied from arterial branches that arise from the ascending aorta. The flow of blood that supplies the heart tissue itself is called the **coronary circulation.** The heart pumps about 380 litres of blood to its own muscle tissue every day.

Heart

The heart is positioned in the thorax underneath the sternum of the rib cage. It has four chambers and is made up primarily of muscle (**Figure 4.1**). The two atria receive blood from the veins and the two ventricles pump blood out into the arteries. The wall of the heart consists of three layers:

1 *Fibrous pericardium* – surrounds the heart giving it support and anchoring it to the diaphragm.
2 *Myocardium* – consists of muscle cells and forms the bulk of the wall of each chamber. This is much thicker in the wall of the left ventricle than the right and, therefore, enables it to develop greater pressure when it contracts. Specialized cells in this layer behave very similarly to nerve cells, generating and transmitting impulses. These cells include the sino-atrial node cells, atrio-ventricular node cells and Purkinje fibres.
3 *Endocardium* – consists of connective tissue, blood vessels and nerves, and forms the innermost layer.

(The septum, the wall separating the right and left sides of the heart, prevents blood passing from one side to the other. The atria and ventricles are separated by dense fibrous tissue.)

Valves

The mitral and tricuspid valves are the valves between the atria and ventricles on the left and right sides of the heart respectively. During ventricular contraction the valve cusps are forced together, closing off the opening and preventing blood from re-entering the atria. The aortic and pulmonary valves

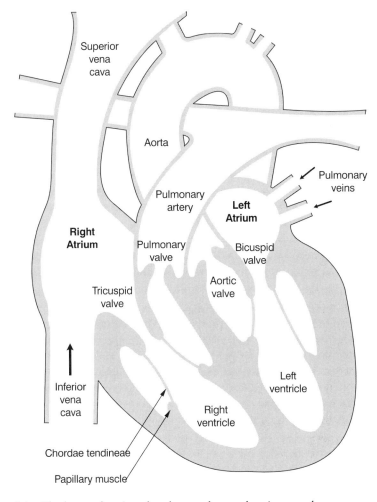

Figure 4.1 – The heart, showing chambers, valves and major vessels

are at the exits of the left and right ventricles. They are called semilunar valves because of their shape. The openings between the veins and the atria are without valves. Therefore, some blood can be forced backwards into the veins and forward into the ventricles when the atria contract.

Cardiac cycle

A single cardiac cycle is the time between the start of one heartbeat and the beginning of the next. It, therefore, includes alternating periods of contraction and relaxation. For each of the heart chambers the cardiac cycle can be divided into two phases. During contraction, or systole, the chamber contracts and blood is pushed into an adjacent chamber or arterial trunk. Diastole follows systole. During diastole, the chamber fills with blood and prepares for the next cardiac cycle. The pressure within each chamber rises during systole and falls during diastole. The valves help to ensure that the blood flows in the correct direction. However, blood will only flow from the first to the second chamber, if the pressure in the first chamber is greater than that of the second. The correct pressure relationship is dependent on the timing of contractions. Blood movement would not occur if the atria and ventricle contacted together.

ELECTROPHYSIOLOGY

The excess of positively charged ions outside the cell membrane, and the slight excess of negatively charged ions inside the cell, causes the inside of a cell membrane to have a slight negative charge with respect to the outside. This unequal distribution of charges is due to the difference in permeability of the cell membrane to the differently charged ions. The positive and negatively charged ions, although separated by a cell membrane, are attracted to one another. A **potential difference** exists when positive and negative ions are held apart. If not separated by a cell membrane, the opposite charges would rush together. The potential difference across a cell membrane is referred to as the **transmembrane potential**. The **volt** is the unit of measurement for potential difference. The transmembrane potential in an undisturbed cell is the **resting potential**. Each cell type has a characteristic resting potential. The normal resting potential is negative. This is because the interior of the cell contains abundant negatively charged proteins, which cannot cross the cell membrane. At the normal resting potential there is a slow leakage of sodium into the cell and a diffusion of potassium out of the cell. A cell expends energy to maintain its resting potential. The sodium–potassium exchange pump stabilizes the resting potential by ejecting sodium ions from within the cell membrane and reclaiming potassium ions from the extracellular fluid.

Membrane channels enable ions to cross the cell membrane. **Passive** and **active** sodium and potassium channels exist. **Leak** or passive channels are always open and are important in maintaining the normal resting potential. Active or **gated** channels open or close in relation to specific stimuli. Three classes of gated channels exist: **chemical-, voltage- or mechanically regulated**. Voltage-regulated channels are characteristic of areas of excitable membrane, i.e. a membrane capable of generating and conducting an **action potential**, e.g. cardiac muscle cells. Voltage-regulated channels open or close in response to changes in the transmembrane potential. The opening of voltage-regulated sodium channels is responsible for the generation of an action potential.

Graded potentials are changes in transmembrane potential that cannot spread far from the site of stimulation. When a membrane is exposed to a chemical that opens chemically regulated sodium channels, sodium ions enter the cell. The arrival of additional positive charges shifts the transmembrane potential towards 0 mV[1] This is called depolarization. The depolarization of surrounding membrane follows the movement of sodium ions across the cell membrane at one location. During this time extracellular sodium ions move towards open channels, replacing those that enter the cell. This is called a **local current**. The number of sodium channels opened by the chemical stimulus is directly proportional to the change in transmembrane potential, and the area affected by the local current. The more channels open the greater the depolarization. When the chemical stimulus is removed the transmembrane potential soon returns to normal. Repolarization is the process of restoring the normal resting potential.

Action potentials are changes in the transmembrane potential that spread across an entire excitable membrane. A graded potential initiates an action potential. A graded potential is large enough to bring an area of excitable membrane to **threshold.** Voltage-regulated sodium channels are opened and allow sodium ions to flood into the cell. There is rapid depolarization. When an action potential is stimulated, it propagates over the entire surface of the excitable membrane. During **repolarization,** sodium channels close, potassium channels open and potassium ions move out of the cell. Finally, all voltage-regulated channels close, and the membrane is back to its resting state.

For a certain period after an action potential begins the membrane will not respond to another stimulus. This is called the **refractory period**. In the **absolute refractory period** the cell will not respond regardless of how strong the stimulus is. An action potential in a cardiac muscle cell differs from that in a skeletal muscle cell due to the presence of a plateau stage between rapid depolarization and repolarization. The plateau represents calcium ion entry via slow calcium channels and prolongs the action potential. The period of active muscle cell contraction continues until the plateau ends. The absolute refractory period continues until relaxation of the cardiac muscle cell is under way. This prevents tetany occurring in cardiac muscle, which would be fatal, as a heart in tetany cannot pump blood.

Conduction system of the heart

During a single heartbeat, the entire heart contracts in a coordinated manner. Thus blood flows in the right direction at the proper time. Contractile cells, and the conducting system, are the cardiac muscle cells involved in a normal heartbeat. Gap junctions connect all heart muscle cells, including the cells of the conduction system, to each other. These gap junctions make it easier for impulses to spread between adjacent cells. So, immediately after a heart cell depolarizes, the cells around it depolarize. In this way, a wave of excitation and contraction spreads over the entire heart.

The conducting system includes:

1   *Sino-atrial (SA) node* – found in the wall of the right atrium.
2   *Atrioventricular (AV) node* – found at the junction between the atria and the ventricles.
3   *Conducting cells* – connect the two nodes and distribute the contractile stimulus throughout the myocardium. Conducting cells in the atria are in the internodal pathway. Ventricular conducting cells include those in the AV bundle, bundle branches and Purkinje fibres. These cells distribute the stimulus to the ventricular myocardium (**Figure 4.2**).

The cells of the conducting system cannot maintain a stable resting potential. As soon as repolarization has occurred, the membrane gradually drifts towards threshold. This rate of spontaneous depolarization varies in

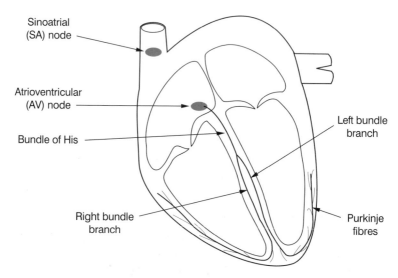

Figure 4.2 – The conduction system of the heart

different portions of the conducting system. It is fastest at the SA node. Cells of the AV node depolarize more slowly and normally most cells of the AV bundle, bundle branches and Purkinje fibres do not depolarize spontaneously. The SA node establishes heart rate as it reaches threshold first.

The SA node contains pacemaker cells, which establish heart rate. The stimulus then crosses the surface of the atria to the AV node. This takes 50 msec. At the AV node, there is a delay of 100 msec and atrial contraction begins. The time elapsed is 150 msec. The connection between the AV node and the AV bundle, or bundle of His, is the only electrical connection between the atria and the ventricles. From the AV bundle, impulses pass through the right and left bundle branches. The left bundle branch is much larger than the right bundle branch. After extending to the apex of the heart, both bundle branches turn out under the endocardial surface. Impulses are then passed on to the Purkinje fibres (time elapsed is 175 msec). The impulses are relayed through the ventricular myocardium. Atrial contraction is complete. Ventricular contraction begins. At this point the total time elapsed is 225 msec.[1]

The normal rhythm of the heart is disturbed if the conducting pathways are damaged. If the SA or internodal pathways are damaged, the AV node will take over. The heart will beat at a slower rate. If a conducting cell or ventricular muscle cell generates an action potential more rapidly than the SA or AV node, then this is called an ectopic pacemaker. This will bypass the conducting system and disrupt the timing of ventricular contraction. This will result in a reduction of the efficiency of the heart, and may be diagnosed with an electrocardiogram.

The Electrocardiogram

Electrodes attached to the surface of the body can detect the electrical changes associated with muscle contraction. An electrocardiogram is a surface recording of the electrical activity of the heart represented graphically. An electrocardiogram can be undertaken for a number of reasons, including:

1 Detection of heart rhythm disturbances
2 Provision of a baseline reading of the electrical activity of the heart
3 Determination of the effects of drugs, e.g. Digoxin
4 Identification of diseases of the conduction system
5 Detection of atrial and ventricular hypertrophy

6 Detection of myocardial infarction or ischaemia
7 Detection of the origin of an arrhythmia
8 Detection of pericarditis
9 Detection of electrolyte imbalance
10 Evaluation of the effectiveness of a cardiac pacemaker

It is important that the ECG is not used in isolation, but in conjunction with an examination of the patient. When taking an ECG, recordings are made from electrodes placed on different parts of the body. Each of the electrode systems is referred to as a lead. Recordings can be taken from limb leads, when electrodes are placed on the arms and legs, or from chest leads, when electrodes are placed on the chest. The limb leads are labelled I, II and III and the chest leads as V_{1-6}. Augmented limb leads are labelled as aV_1, aV_r and aV_f to donate left and right arm and foot.

The limb leads are bipolar, i.e. the electrical activity is monitored at two sites and compared by the recording equipment. By convention, the right arm is a negative pole, the left arm is a positive pole (except in lead III, where it is negative), and the left leg is a positive pole. Lead I records the potential between the right arm and the left arm. Lead II records the potential between the right arm and the left leg (when a patient is placed on a cardiac monitor the electrodes are normally placed in such a position to record this potential). Lead III records the potential between the left arm and left leg. The chest leads are unipolar, monitoring activity at one site. The lead placed on the chest is the positive pole and the limb leads form the negative pole. The augmented limb leads are unipolar and compare the differences between a given point and zero (**Figure 4.3**).

Impulses travel from negative to a positive pole. The impulses travelling towards the positive pole give a positive deflection on the ECG graph paper. The shape of the ECG varies, depending on the lead used, i.e. the waves are there, and their timing the same, but their shape and size are different. The recordings taken from a patient on a cardiac monitor, are normally taken from limb lead II.

From an electrical viewpoint, the heart can be thought of as having two chambers, the atria and the ventricles. The muscle mass of the atria is small. Therefore, their contraction and accompanying electrical changes are small. When the ventricles contract, there is a large deflection on the ECG. **Figure 4.4** is a diagram of the basic ECG waveform.

All ECG machines run at a standard rate, each using paper with standard squares. The horizontal axis represents time.

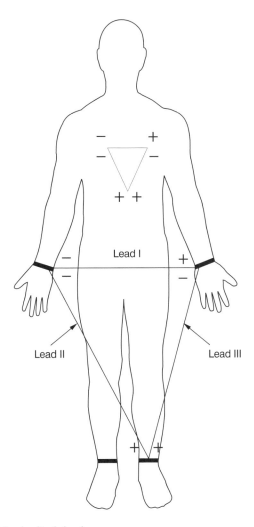

Figure 4.3 – The bipolar limb leads

1   One small square = 0.04 seconds
2   One large square = 0.2 seconds

The vertical axis represents voltage/magnitude:

1   One small square = 1 mm
2   One large square = 5 mm or 0.5 mV

It is important that the ECG machine is standardized, 1 mV giving a deflection of 10 mm (1 cm).

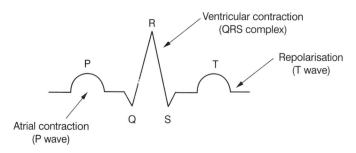

Figure 4.4 – The basic ECG waveform

Recording an ECG

Before attempting to record an ECG, the nurse must be familiar with the ECG machine and how to operate it. This will help to prevent an incorrect recording and in turn prevent an incorrect diagnosis and time wastage. The patient should be lying down and relaxed to reduce electrical interference from skeletal muscle. A good electrical contact is required, therefore, before attaching the electrodes. It may be necessary to wipe the skin with a spirit wipe and remove excess hair. The bipolar limb electrodes and unipolar chest electrodes should be correctly positioned (**Figure 4.5**). The electrodes will usually be labelled or colour-coded to assist in this process.

Before commencing recording, check that the machine is set at the correct paper speed (usually 25 mm/second) and that the calibration mark has been made such that 10 mm = 1 mV (wave height can then be readily converted into a more meaningful voltage).

Recognition of cardiac rhythms

The following describes a number of easy steps involved in the recognition of cardiac rhythm.[2]

QRS rate

The QRS complex represents ventricular depolarization. The QRS rate is classified as:

1   Normal – 60–100/minute
2   Bradycardic (slow) – < 60/minute
3   Severely bradycardic – < 40/minute
4   Tachycardic (fast) – between 150 and 200/minute

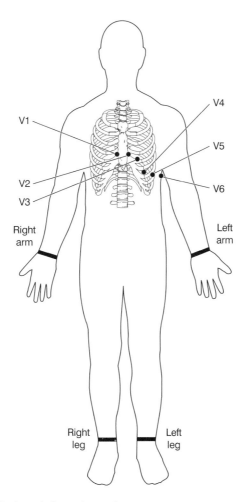

Figure 4.5 – ECG limb and chest electrodes

Heart rate can be calculated by counting the number of large 5 mm squares between consecutive R waves, and then divide this number into 300. This is demonstrated in **Table 4.1**.

QRS rhythm

By mapping out each of the R waves, it is possible to identify whether the QRS rhythm is regular or irregular.

Are there any pauses present? (A pause > 3 seconds requires rapid investigation as there is a risk of asystole).

Table 4.1 – *R-R interval and heart rate*

No. of 5 mm squares between R waves.	Heart rate (beats per min.)
1	300
1.5	200
2	150
3	100
4	75
5	60
6	50
7	45
8	40
9	35
10	30

QRS duration

Is the QRS broad or narrow? It should normally be 0.12 seconds (three small squares or less). Any abnormality of conduction takes longer and causes widening of the QRS complex. Widening of the QRS complex generally occurs when the speed of impulses are either triggered from an ectopic focus or fail to take the correct route. It takes longer for the spread of impulses to depolarize the myocardium, giving rise to a broad QRS complex.

Atrial activity

The 'P' wave represents normal atrial activity.

1 Are the P waves absent?
2 Are they all the same shape and morphology?
3 Is the pattern irregular?
4 Is there any atrial fibrillation?
5 Are there any atrial flutter waves (saw toothed in shape and at a rate of 300 per minute)?

Atrio-ventricular relationship

1 Is there 1:1 conduction (i.e. one P wave to one QRS complex), or is it 2:1 or 3:1?
2 Is the P-R interval normal, i.e. between 0.12 and 0.2 seconds (three-to-five small squares) and a constant length throughout the rhythm?

Abnormal cardiac rhythms

The conduction pathway and normal rhythm of the heart can be damaged in a number of ways, including:

1   Mechanical distortion
2   Ischaemia
3   Infection
4   Inflammation

The resulting deficit is called a heart block. In first-degree heart block the AV node and proximal part of the AV bundle slows the passage of impulses. A pause appears between the atrial and ventricular contraction. However, the heart rhythm is regular and a QRS complex follows each P wave. In mild second-degree heart block an occasional skipped beat may be seen. If the delay lasts long enough the ventricles will follow every second atrial beat. This pattern of 'atria, atria-ventricles, atria, atria-ventricles' is known as a 2:1 block. It is possible for an individual to develop a three-to-one or even a four-to-one block. During third-degree heart block or complete heart block the conduction pathway no longer functions. Although the atria and the ventricles beat, their activity is not synchronized. The atria follow the pace set by the SA node beating about 70–80 times per minute, and the ventricles follow the pace set by the AV node, beating about 40–60 times per minute.

Premature atrial contractions (PAC) can occur in healthy individuals. In PAC the normal atrial rhythm is interrupted by a surprise contraction. Stress, drugs and caffeine can all increase the incidence of PAC. In paroxysmal atrial tachycardia (PAT) a flurry of atrial activity is stimulated by a premature atrial contraction. The ventricles keep pace with the atria and the heart rate can be 180 beats per minute. During atria flutter the atria contract in a coordinated manner with frequent contractions. In atrial fibrillation the impulses travel over the atria at about 500 beats per minute. The walls of the atria quiver as opposed to producing an organized contraction. The ventricular rate remains within normal limits as they cannot keep pace with the atrial rate. Both these conditions can go unnoticed and are not considered very dangerous unless they are prolonged or associated with other cardiac damage, e.g. coronary artery disease. By contrast ventricular arrhythmias can be serious and even fatal.

As the heart's conduction system functions in one direction only, ventricular arrhythmias are not linked to atrial activity. Premature ventricular contractions (PVC) occur when a Purkinje cell or ventricular myocardial cell depolarizes to threshold and triggers a premature contraction. The cell causing this is called the ectopic pacemaker. Ventricular tachycardia (VT) often precedes ventricular fibrillation (VF), the most serious arrhythmia. This condition is fatal as the heart stops pumping blood. Impulses are travelling from cell to cell and around the ventricular walls. A normal rhythm cannot occur because the ventricular cells are stimulating each other at such a rapid rate. A defibrillator is used to restore normal cardiac rhythm (see **Chapter 5**). It is very important not to diagnose asystole as fine VF. Asystole means there is no spontaneous electrical cardiac activity. There is an absence of ventricular activity and heart rate is zero.

References

1. Martini, F.H. *Fundamentals of Anatomy and Physiology* (4th edition). 1998; Prentice Hall International.

2. Hampden, J.R. *The ECG Made Easy* (4th edition). 1992; Edinburgh: Churchill Livingstone.

Suggested Reading

1. Hampden, J.R. *The ECG Made Easy* (4th edition). 1992; Edinburgh: Churchill Livingstone.

2. Hampden, J.R. *The ECG in Practice* (2nd edition). 1992; Edinburgh: Churchill Livingstone.

3. Houghton A.R., Gray D. *Making Sense of the ECG* (2nd edition). 1997; London: Arnold.

Review questions

1. Where does the pulmonary circulation carry blood to and from?
2. Where does the systemic circulation carry blood to and from?
3. What is the anatomical difference between the right and left ventricle?
4. What do valves prevent?
5. What is the function of the coronary circulation?
6. Where do the coronary arteries originate?
7. Starting at the vena cava, describe the direction of blood flow through the heart.

8. The left atrioventricular valve has two names, what are they?

9. What determines the resting potential of a neurone?

10. The cell membrane contains active (gated) channels and passive (leak) channels. Describe the functions of these channels.

11. Name two types of gated channels.

12. When would an action potential appear?

13. What is the role of the sodium–potassium exchange pump?

14. What are the two classes of cardiac muscle cells involved in the normal heartbeat?

15. What is the route of conduction of an electrical impulse from the SA node to the ventricles?

16. Do cardiac muscle cells need neural or hormonal stimulation to contract?

17. Which cells establish the rate of contraction?

18. Identify the following rhythms (**Figure 4.6**)

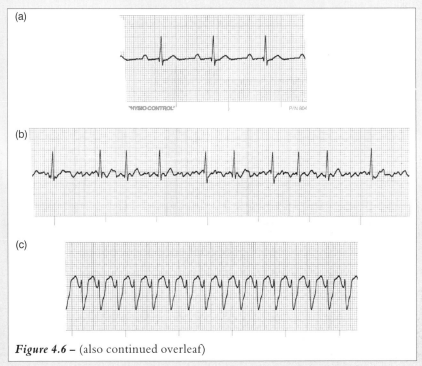

(a)

(b)

(c)

Figure 4.6 – (also continued overleaf)

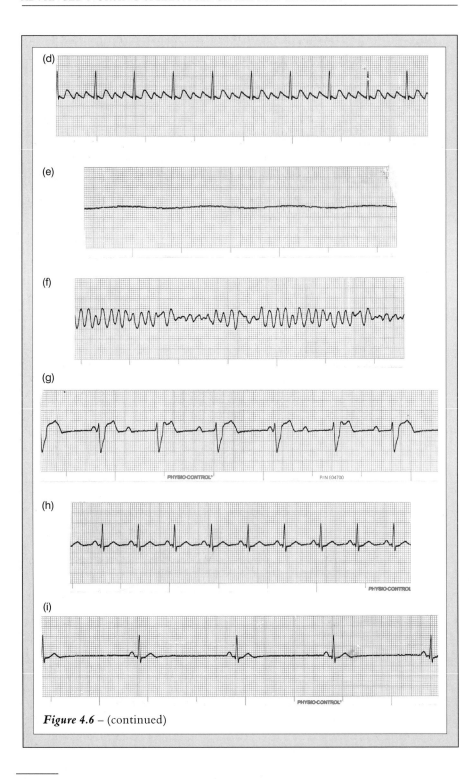

Figure 4.6 – (continued)

Review questions – answers

1. To and from the lungs

2. The rest of the body

3. The right ventricle is thin in comparison with the left ventricle, which has a very thick muscular wall

4. The regurgitation of blood

5. To meet the high oxygen and nutrient demands of the cardiac muscle cells

6. The base of the ascending aorta

7. Vena cava – right atrium – right ventricle – pulmonary circulation (pulmonary artery, pulmonary vein) – left atrium – left ventricle – aorta

8. Mitral valve and bicuspid valve

9. The membrane's permeability to potassium

10. Channels through which ions are able to pass to enter or leave a cell

11. Chemical, voltage and mechanically regulated

12. When a region of excitable membrane depolarizes to threshold

13. Maintain ion concentration (inside and outside the cell membrane) within acceptable limits

14. Contractile cells and conducting system

15. SA node – across atria – AV node – bundle of His – right and left bundle branches – Purkinje fibres – left ventricle

16. No

17. Pacemaker cells in the SA node.

18. (a) First-degree heart block

    (b) Atrial fibrillation

    (c) Ventricular tachycardia

    (d) Atrial flutter

    (e) Asystole

    (f) Ventricular fibrillation

    (g) Complete heart block

    (h) Sinus tachycardia

    (i) Sinus bradycardia

5

DEFIBRILLATION

The key factors that influence the chance of a successful outcome following cardiopulmonary arrest include:

- Access to the emergency medical system

- The commencement of basic life support (BLS) within 4 min

- Defibrillation within 8 min for ventricular fibrillation or pulseless ventricular tachycardia

- The early administration of advanced care, i.e. drugs and endotracheal intubation[1]

Manual defibrillation relies on immediate arrhythmia recognition and has historically been the responsibility of medical staff or specialist critical care nurses. However, with the advent of the automated external defibrillation (AED), nurses not trained in rhythm recognition and manual defibrillation are increasingly undertaking this practice. A review of normal cardiac conduction was presented in **Chapter 4**. Here, this knowledge is applied to the procedure for defibrillation.

VENTRICULAR FIBRILLATION AND PULSELESS VENTRICULAR TACHYCARDIA

Defibrillation is the delivery of an electrical current to the heart muscle and is the most effective treatment for ventricular fibrillation (VF) and pulseless ventricular tachycardia. VF is life threatening. It is a rapid and irregular rhythm resulting from uncoordinated depolarization throughout the myocardium. The ventricles cannot contract and blood is not pumped from the heart. The ventricles actually appear to quiver. VF is commonly associated with coronary artery disease and myocardial infarction (particularly during the first 48 hours following the infarction). It can also occur during an electrical shock, drowning, acid–base disturbances and drug toxicity.[2]

As described in **Chapter 4**, the PR interval on the electrocardiogram (ECG) (**Figure 4.4**) represents the conduction delay between the atria and the ventricles. The QRS complex represents ventricular depolarization. The first half of the T-wave on the ECG is known as the refractory or vulnerable period and lasts for about 30 milliseconds (**Figure 5.1**). If a patient suffers from myocardial ischaemia the vulnerable period may extend to include the upslope of the T-wave and persist over the apex of this wave.[3]

The tissues involved in the conduction system and the majority of the myocardial cells can generate electrical impulses. This is known as automaticity. The heart, therefore, has many potential pacemakers. These 'ectopic' pacemakers can fire prematurely and cause a contraction even if the sino-atrial (SA) node is functioning correctly. If, in a healthy heart, ectopic impulses interrupt the cardiac cycle during the vulnerable period, this does not normally cause a problem and the SA node regains control. However, in

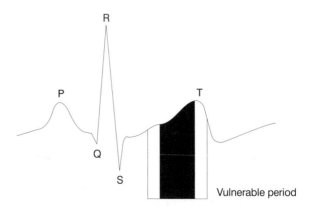

Figure 5.1 – A basic ECG waveform showing the refractory or vulnerable period

a diseased heart, VF might be stimulated. VF will not correct itself and defibrillation must be performed. The period before commencement of defibrillation is critical to the patient's chance of survival.[4] Ideally, this should be no more than 90 seconds as hypoxic injury to the brain will begin to occur after this period.[5]

Defibrillation

The defibrillator is designed to deliver an electrical impulse to the patient's chest via paddle electrodes or disposable defibrillation electrodes. Defibrillation may be manually operated or automated, i.e. AED.

Manual defibrillation requires both knowledge and skills in relation to rhythm recognition. The operator must identify whether defibrillation is indicated. The shock strength is set manually on the defibrillator and the defibrillator is charged. Following the placement of the electrode paddles on the patient's chest an electrical current is delivered.

By comparison, arrhythmia analysis and preparation for defibrillation is automated with AED. Following recognition of a cardiac arrest, two large adhesive electrodes must be attached to the patient's chest. These electrodes monitor the cardiac rhythm and also defibrillate. The AED charges to the predetermined level and indicates when to discharge the current if it has identified that the rhythm is appropriate. This enables early defibrillation to be undertaken in a variety of settings by staff untrained in rhythm recognition and manual defibrillation. AED may be fully or semiautomatic. Whereas a fully automatic device detects a shockable rhythm, charges and delivers a shock (following the operator pressing a button on the machine), a semiautomatic or 'shock advisory' device advises the user to deliver a shock and may charge automatically.

Defibrillation can be applied internally through the patient's open chest or externally through the chest wall. Two paddle positions are recommended:[6]

- Anteriolateral position
- Anterior-posterior position

Anteriolateral position

In this position the sternum paddle is placed on the patient's upper right chest to the right of the sternum below the clavicle. The apex paddle is placed on the patient's lower left chest over the cardiac apex, to the left of the nipple in the mid-axillary line, i.e. the V_4–V_5 position in an ECG (**Figure 5.2**). This position is used most frequently because the anterior chest is more accessible.[7]

Anterior-posterior position

The anterior paddle is placed over the cardiac apex just to the left of the left sternal border, and the posterior paddle is placed on the patient's left posterior chest beneath the scapula and lateral to the spine[7] (**Figure 5.3**).

During defibrillation the chest receives a current that depolarizes a majority of ventricular cells. If, when this current is removed, a critical mass (75–90%) of the cells is in the same phase, i.e. recovery or **repolarization**, defibrillation occurs.[8] The SA node or other intrinsic pacemaker can then gain control. The time that the patient is in VF is a factor, which is directly related to whether an intrinsic pacemaker can do this.[9] Other factors that affect the intrinsic pacemaker gaining control include myocardial function, oxygenation and acid–base balance of the heart muscle.[9]

The operational factors that affect the success of defibrillation include the time period from fibrillation to defibrillation, the position of the defibrillator paddles, energy level and transthoracic impedence (TTI).

Time

The faster that defibrillation can be instituted from fibrillation, the greater the likelihood of a positive outcome.[2] If the delivery of defibrillation from

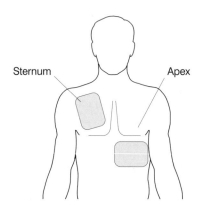

Figure 5.2 – Sternum – Apex or anteriolateral placement

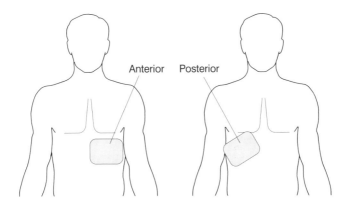

Figure 5.3 – Anterior – Posterior placement

fibrillation is greater than 8 minutes there is a risk of neurological damage. The chance of patient survival is greatly decreased if this delay is more than 10 minutes.[10]

Paddle position

The defibrillation paddles must be placed so that the ventricles are in the pathway of the electrical current. Bone is a poor conductor of electricity; therefore, paddles should not be placed over the sternum.

Energy requirement

The European Resuscitation and Resuscitation Council (UK)[11] recommend that for conventional monophasic defibrillators the first shock is 200 J; the second shock, if the first is unsuccessful, should also be 200 J. Subsequent shocks should be 360 J. However, newer defibrillators using biphasic waveforms may require less energy. Therefore, it is recommended[11] to 'defibrillate × 3 as necessary' (**Figure 5.4**). There is no need to check for a pulse in between each and every shock. It is currently recommended that a pulse check is only required if, following a defibrillator shock, the cardiac rhythm changes to one compatible with a cardiac output.[11]

Transthoracic impedence (TTI)

TTI is the resistance created by structures in the thorax to the electrical current as it passes through the chest. TTI combined with shock energy

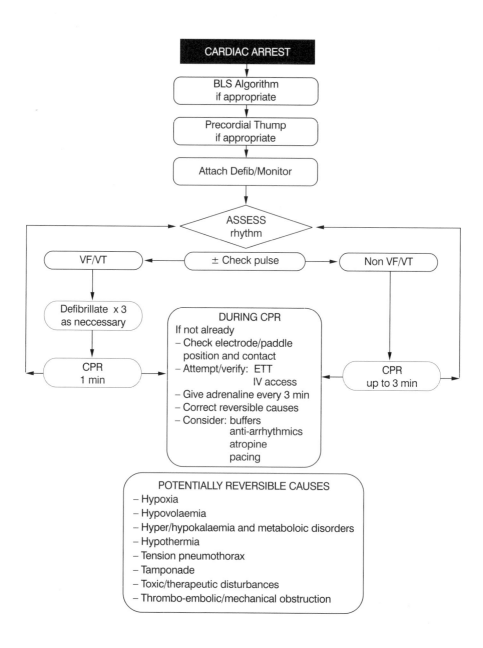

Figure 5.4 – The algorthm for advanced life support
(© Resuscitation Council UK 1997)[11]

determines the amount of current that actually reaches the heart.[12] If defibrillation is undertaken correctly, this will help to overcome TTI. TTI is affected by the following variables.

Paddle size

Larger paddles lower the resistance to current flow, so allowing a greater amount of current to reach the heart. This increases the possibility of successful defibrillation and decreases the probability of myocardial damage. However, paddles must not be so large that they are in contact with one another or do not adhere to the walls of the chest.[7] Recommended paddle size for adults is 8–13 cm in diameter.[4]

Skin–paddle interface

The skin is not a good conductor of electricity. A material such as electrode gel or gel pads at the skin paddle interface is necessary. If this is not used the amount of current that reaches the heart during defibrillation is decreased. Furthermore, the skin may become burned.

Shocks and time between shocks

Following the initial defibrillation attempt TTI decreases by 8%. However, with further attempts TTI is decreased by 4%.[12] The level of decrease in TTI is dependent on the period between shocks. The closer the shocks, the lower the TTI. For a persistent VF it is recommended that 'serial' shocks without removal of defibrillator paddles from the chest between the second and third shocks are administered.[13]

Paddle pressure

By pressing the paddles firmly, contact between the skin and paddle is improved. A pressure of 11 kg (25 lb) on each paddle is recommended.[6] This pressure also brings the paddles closer together and causes a decrease in the volume of air in the lungs.

Ventilation

Air is a poor conductor of electricity. It is, therefore, recommended that shocks are delivered during full expiration.[14] This reduces the resistance to current flow.

Safety during defibrillation

All personnel should stand clear of the bed and patient immediately before defibrillation. The only contact should be by the defibrillator operator through the defibrillator paddle handles. Gel or defibrillation pads should be applied before charging the defibrillator. Care must be taken not to use too much gel, and paddles should be correctly positioned. If gel becomes continuous with the paddle sites or comes into contact with the paddle handles, this provides a means by which a stray current can pass.[7]

Environmental hazards such as wet surroundings or clothing should be removed. There should also be no electrical leakage from other electrical equipment in the surrounding area. As oxygen supports combustion, oxygen administration devices should be removed from the bed during defibrillation.

References

1. Cummins, R.O., Ornato, J.P., Thies, W.H., Pepe, P.E. Improving survival from sudden cardiac arrest: the 'chain of survival' concept. A statement for health professionals from the advanced cardiac life support committee and emergency cardiac care committee of the American Heart Association. *Circulation* 1991; 83: 1832–1847.

2. Cummins, R.O. Defibrillation. *Emergency Medicine Clinics of North America* 1988; 6: 217–240.

3. American National Standards Institute (ANSI)/Association for the Advancement of Medical Instrumentation (AAMI). 1989. *Cardiac defibrillator devices.* DF2.

4. European Resuscitation Council *Guidelines for Resuscitation.* 1998; Antwerp: ERC.

5. Colquhoun, M.C., Handley, A.J., Evans, T.R. *ABC of Resuscitation.* (3rd edition). 1995; London: BMJ.

6. American Heart Association *Textbook of Advanced Cardiac Life Support* (2nd edition). 1987; AHA.

7. Crocket, P.J., Droppert, B.M., Higgins, S.E. *Defibrillation – what you should know* (3rd edition). 1991; Physio-Control Corporation.

8. Zhou, X., Daubert, J.P., Wolf, P.D. *et al.* Size of the critical mass for defibrillation. Abstracts of the 62nd scientific sessions of the American Heart Association. *Circulation* 1980; 80 (suppl. 11): 11–531.

9. Cummins, R.O. Defibrillation. *Emergency Medicine Clinics of North America* 1988; 6: 217–240.

10. Weaver, W.D., Cobb, L.A., Hallstrom, A.P. *et al*. Factors influencing survival after out-of-hospital cardiac arrest. *Journal of the American College of Cardiology* 1986; 7: 752–757.

11. European Resuscitation Council. Guidelines for Adult Advanced Life Support. *Resuscitation* 1988; 37(2).

12. Kerber, R.E., Grayzel, J., Hoyt, R. *et al* Transthoracic resistance in human defibrillation. Influence of body weight, chest size, serial shocks, paddle size and paddle contract pressure. *Circulation* 1981; 63: 676–682.

13. Dahl, C.F., Ewy, G.A., Ewy, M.D. *et al*. Transthoracic impedance to direct current discharge; effect of repeated countershocks. *Medical Instrumentation* 1976; 10: 151–154.

14. Sirna, S.J., Ferguson, D.W., Charbonnier, F. *et al*. Factors affecting transthoracic impedance during electrical cardioversion. *American Journal of Cardiology* 1988; 62: 1048–1052.

Review questions

1. During which arrhythmias would you administer defibrillation?

2. When might VF occur?

3. What is the ventricular refractory or vulnerable period?

4. What are the two paddle positions recommended for defibrillation?

5. What happens to the ventricular cells during depolarization?

6. Name three factors that influence the success of defibrillation.

7. What is meant by TTI?

Review questions – answers

1. Ventricular fibrillation and pulseless ventricular tachycardia

2. Electrical shock, drug toxicity, acid–base disturbances, drowning, following a myocardial infarction

3. First half of the T-wave on an ECG – the muscle fibres are repolarizing and returning to the resting state

4. Anteriolateral, anterior-posterior

5. Depolarization

6. Time, paddle position, TTI

7. Structures within the thorax that cause resistance to the passage of an electrical current

6

NUTRITIONAL ASSESSMENT AND ENTERAL TUBE FEEDING

Malnutrition can complicate illness, prolong hospital stay, and increase mortality and the likelihood of readmission[1]. In order that appropriate nutritional support can be provided, it is of paramount importance that healthcare professionals can identify those individuals at risk of malnourishment and those already malnourished. An overview of the anatomy and physiology of the digestive system is first presented. Malnutrition in the hospitalized patient and nutritional screening and assessment are then discussed. Finally, enteral feeding as a method of nutritional support is considered.

APPLIED ANATOMY AND PHYSIOLOGY

The digestive system

The digestive tract includes the oral cavity, oesophagus, stomach and intestines (**Figure 6.1**). It is basically a hollow muscular tube, mucosal epithelium lining the inner surface, and circular and longitudinal muscle

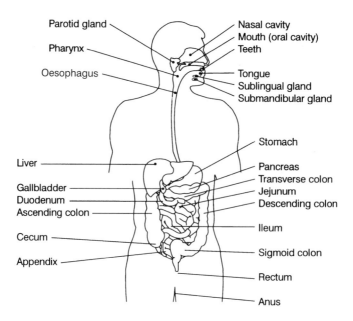

Figure 6.1 – Organs of the digestive system and related structures

comprising the walls. The mucosa forming the inner lining of the tract is supplied with a rich network of blood vessels, nerve fibres and endocrine cells. Epithelial cells (specialized for both absorption and secretion depending on their location in the digestive tract) cover this mucosal layer. The serosa is a layer of connective tissue covering the tract on the outside.

In the mouth, food is broken down to small pieces and worked upon by digestive enzymes in the saliva. After chewing, the food is passed along the digestive tract by muscular action and mixed with further enzymes. These enzymes digest carbohydrates, fats and proteins. The end products of digestion include glucose, amino acids, fats, glycerol and fatty acids. These are absorbed through the gut wall and transported to the cells by the blood stream. The movement and mixing of food in the digestive tract, and its elimination, is brought about primarily by the contractions of smooth muscle. Striated muscle, however, is involved in the mouth, pharynx and upper oesophagus, and external anal sphincter.

Oesophagus

The oesophagus is a thin-walled tube attaching the pharynx to the stomach. It consists of striated muscle at the top and smooth muscle at the bottom.

When food is swallowed, the sphincter in the upper portion of the oesophagus relaxes and peristalsis propels food through the oesophagus. If food particles remain in the oesophagus following this wave of peristalsis, another wave of peristalsis is stimulated which sweeps food through into the stomach. The sphincter at the lower end of the stomach prevents the regurgitation of food from the stomach back into the oesophagus. The final few centimetres of the osesophagus are actually in the abdominal cavity. Therefore, when abdominal pressure increase, e.g. when coughing, this terminal section of the oesophagus is compressed and stomach contents are not forced to enter into the oesophagus.[2]

STOMACH

The stomach is divided into the fundus, body and pyloric antrum (**Figure 6.2**). The fundus and body are relatively thin walled and act as a reservoir for ingested food. When food is swallowed the muscle layers relax. If this relaxation does not occur, a person feels ill very quickly after only a few mouthfuls

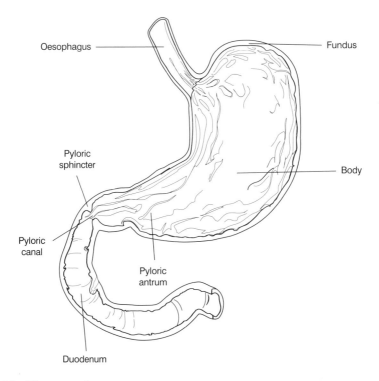

Figure 6.2 – The stomach

of food.[2] The pyloric antrum has thick walls and strong waves of contraction occur during the digestion of a meal. The food is mixed with gastric juices and then passes from the stomach to the duodenum via the pyloric canal. A band of smooth muscle circles this canal and is called the pyloric sphincter.

Following ingestion of a meal, the body and fundus distend. Ripples of contraction (occurring about three times a minute) then begin in the middle of the stomach forcing the food towards the pyloric antrum and pyloric canal. These peristaltic waves occur about three times a minute and become greater in intensity as they reach the pyloric canal.[2] Therefore, every 20 seconds a portion of the stomach contents is pushed towards the pyloric canal. It is then propelled into the intestine. As the pyloric sphincter contracts, the mixture is pushed back into the body of the stomach. This mixture becomes reduced into chyme, a semi-fluid substance and each minute, 6–10 ml of chyme is emptied into the intestine.[2]

SMALL INTESTINE

The small intestine is about 6 metres in length and is divided into the duodenum (the section closest to the stomach), the jejunum and the ileum (the last segment of the small intestine). Nearly all the nutrient absorption occurs in this structure. Segmentation rather than peristalsis is seen in the small intestine. As a result of the contraction of circular muscle at several points along this structure, the small intestine is divided into a number of sacs. The circular muscles then contract at different places and this causes the chyme to be pushed backwards and forwards and mixed with digestive enzymes. Longitudinal muscles also contract and relax and massage the contents of the intestine. The movement of chyme through the small intestine is very slow. This allows digestion and absorption of food. 3–4 hours following a meal, food residues arrive at the end of the small intestine.

LARGE INTESTINE

The large intestine is about 1.5 m long and 7.5 cm wide (**Figure 6.3**). It is comprised of three parts: caecum, colon and rectum. The ascending colon travels up the right side of the abdomen towards the liver. It turns at the hepatic flexure and becomes the transverse colon. It then turns down the left side of the abdomen at the splenic flexure and becomes the descending colon. This then becomes the pelvic colon, the rectum and finally the anus.

Each day about 500 ml of food material, or chyme, enter the caecum. The longitudinal muscle of the large intestine forms three strips. These muscles are not as long as the colon itself. Therefore, the wall of the intestine becomes puckered and pouches called haustra are formed. Peristaltic movements of the large intestine tend to be slow and non-propulsive. This aids absorption and storage functions. Haustral contractions occurring at intervals of about 30 minutes shuffle the contents of the intestine back and forth. Large contractions, called mass movements, occur three to four times a day. This drives the colonic contents forward for storage in the rectum.

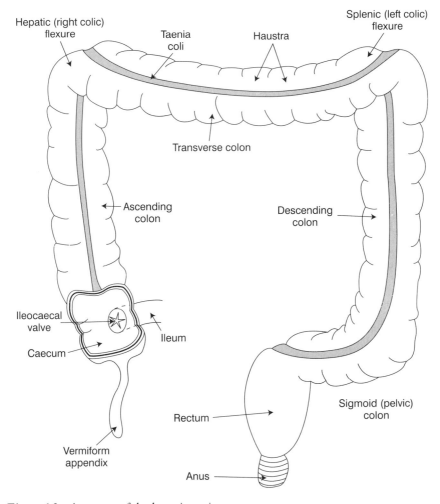

Figure 6.3 – Anatomy of the large intestine

The large intestine actively absorbs sodium from the ascending and transverse colon. This is then followed by the passive absorption of chloride and water. About 350 ml is absorbed from the 500 ml chyme entering the colon, 150 g faecal material then has to be eliminated. This includes 100 g water and 50 g solids. The length of time the food residue remains in the large intestine will determine the amount of water absorbed.

The large intestine also secretes an alkaline mucus. This lubricates the faeces and facilitates their passage through the intestine. The mucus also contains bicarbonate that maintains colonic pH. The mucosa is also protected by the bicarbonate, which neutralizes acids produced by bacterial fermentation.

Malnutrition

Malnutrition may occur as a result of several factors, which include:

- A decreased dietary intake
- An increased dietary requirement
- An impaired ability to absorb or metabolize nutrients[1]

Conditions that may necessitate nutritional support include:

- Patients with swallowing difficulties such as those with motor neurone disease, multiple sclerosis and cerebral vascular accidents
- Patients malnourished on admission to hospital, i.e. before surgery
- Patients with increased nutritional requirements, e.g. wound infections/sepsis, fractures and postoperative patients
- Patients with gastrointestinal disease, e.g. inflammatory bowel disease
- Patients with a chronic condition, e.g. respiratory condition
- Patients with a depressed appetite, e.g. due to cancer, especially during or after chemotherapy or radiotherapy

Undernutrition can complicate illness, delay recovery, potentiate infection, enhance the risk of pressure sores, decrease the rate of wound healing, prolong hospital stay, and increase mortality and the likelihood of readmission.[1] Therefore, it is essential that healthcare professionals undertake nutritional screening and assessment to ensure that nutritional support is provided as soon as possible to those patients at risk.[3,4]

Malnutrition in hospitalized patients

The incidence of malnutrition in hospitalized patients was first reported in both the USA and the UK more than 20 years ago.[5–7] However, undernutrition still remains a significant problem.[1] It has been identified that 40% of those patients admitted to UK hospitals are malnourished and 75% demonstrate adverse changes in their nutritional status on discharge home.[8] It has been suggested that enteral nutrition should be considered in every patient undergoing major surgery.[9]

Malnutrition may be exacerbated by a number of factors including:

- Unappealing meals
- 'Missed meals' due to staff visits at mealtimes
- Psychological factors such as stress and anxiety
- Treatment-related factors such as prolonged fasting
- Drug therapy interfering with food metabolism[1]

Although malnourishment can occur in any patient, certain groups of patients are particularly vulnerable, including:

- The elderly
- Cancer patients
- Patients with respiratory problems
- Patients with gastrointestinal problems
- Unconscious patients[1]

Nutritional screening

Nutritional screening tools exist that enable the practitioner to identify those patients at risk of malnourishment and those already malnourished. The tools each include questions that specifically focus on known risk factors for malnutrition.[10] Commonly, points are scored for each factor. The total score then provides a measurement of risk.

Nutritional assessment

Nutritional assessment involves the use of measures to determine nutritional status.[10] The goals of nutritional assessment have been identified as:

- To identify patients who have or are at risk of developing protein-energy malnutrition, or specific nutrient deficiencies

- To quantify a patient's risk of developing malnutrition-related complications

- To monitor the adequacy of nutritional therapy[11]

Two or three measures are normally used together to assess nutritional status. These measures must be repeated regularly to monitor the effectiveness of nutritional support. Measures include:

- Dietary history

- Clinical examination

- Anthropometric, biochemical and function tests[10]

Nutritional support

Nutritional support aims to correct or prevent any deficiencies and improve the patient's nutritional status. It can be provided by:

- Improved oral nutrition

- Enteral tube feeding, i.e. nasogastric feeding, nasoduodenal feeding, jejunostomy feeding and gastrostomy feeding (percutaneous endoscopic gastrostomy)

- Total parenteral nutrition (TPN)

The most effective route for feeding is via the mouth. If the ability to eat or drink is compromised, the administration of nutrients into the gastrointestinal tract via a tube (enteral nutrition) may then be considered. When normal gastrointestinal function is not present, parenteral nutrition is necessary.

Enteral feeding

Enteral feeding may be used to provide the patient's entire nutritional requirements, or to supplement the diet of an individual unable to take in sufficient oral nutrition. Enteral feeding can be administered via a number of different routes (**Figure 6.4**).

A number of factors must be considered before commencing enteral nutrition, including:

- Access route
- Enteral diet
- Delivery systems
- Method of delivery
- Monitoring
- Complications[12]

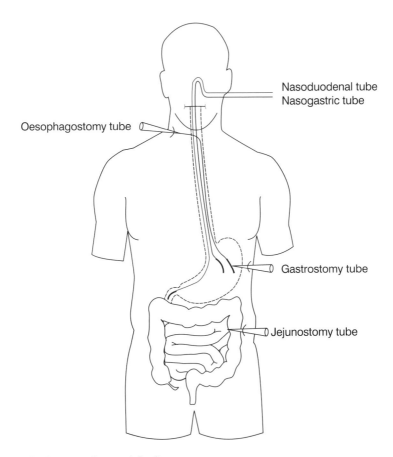

Figure 6.4 – Routes of enteral feeding

Once the decision to commence enteral nutrition has been made, the route of access is primarily dependent upon whether a patient requires short- or long-term feeding.

Nasogastric feeding

It has been identified that the majority of hospitalized patients only require nutritional support for less than 4 weeks.[12] The most effective method of enteral delivery is by fine-bore nasogastric tube (FBT) feeding. FBT should be used whenever possible. These tubes are more comfortable for the patient than wide-bore tubes. They do not interfere with swallowing and oesophageal irritation is less likely. The tubes are generally made from soft polyurethane or silicone elastomer with a diameter of less than 3 mm. Owing to their ability to tolerate gastric secretions, these tubes remain in position longer than PVC tubes which have a lifespan of 10–14 days. Fine-bore tube insertion must be undertaken by staff trained in this technique because of the risk of pneumothorax as a result of an ill-positioned tube. A guide wire facilitates the insertion of the FBT. This guide wire must never be removed and reinserted as it could pierce the FBT and then the oesophagus.[12] Correct positioning of the tube in the stomach can be confirmed by syringe aspiration of gastric contents (pH < 3) and auscultation of the epigastrium. Confirmation of the position of the tube by X-ray is essential if these methods are unsuccessful. X-ray confirmation must always be undertaken in patients with altered consciousness levels, altered cough or gag reflex or in those who are mechanically ventilated.[12] Unplanned removal of FBT is the most common complication that causes an interruption of enteral feeding regimen. This occurs in about 60% of patients and involves accidental or deliberate removal by patients, accidental removal by staff, and the vomiting up of tubes[10]. Fixing the tube to the nose and face with tape and regular examination will keep unplanned removal of tubes to a minimum.[12]

Patients at risk of enteral diet regurgitation or pulmonary aspiration of feed, e.g. the elderly and ventilated patients, should be considered for jejunal or duodenal feeding.[12]

Gastrostomy

FBT feeding is not the ideal route for longer-term feeding, i.e. more than 3–4 weeks. In these situations percutaneous endoscopic gastrostomy (PEG) feeding is often used. This involves the insertion of a gastrostomy tube directly into the stomach through the abdominal wall under endoscopic control using local anaesthesia. PEG tubes are made from polyurethane or silicone and held in position by a flange or inflated balloon. The gastrostomy site is usually cleaned aseptically with normal saline and a sterile dressing applied. The site should also be observed for leakage and infection. A low incidence of minor complications has been found with PEG.

These complications are associated with poor technique or stoma site care, and include leakage, bleeding and local infection.[12]

Administration of enteral feeds

It is important that precautions are taken during the administration of enteral feeding to prevent the development of infection. Patients receiving enteral nutrition are frequently immunocompromised as a result of their malnutrition. Enteral diet contamination may originate from a number of areas (**Table 6.1**) and, where possible, these sources of contamination must be eliminated.

The use of commercially prepared feeds and closed feeding systems greatly reduces the risk of infection. Commercially prepared feeds usually come in 500 ml containers. These containers and the large volume reservoirs available simplify the handling and nursing care required. However, once enteral diets are contaminated they normally provide an ideal medium for bacterial growth. The risk of contamination is increased if feeds need to be diluted or reconstituted. Therefore, sterile gloves should be worn during

Table 6.1 – Sources of contamination during enteral feed administration[12]

- The patient, i.e. an ascending infection of the diet container from the enteral tube via the giving set
- The feed itself
- During the reconstitution or dilution of the feed
- The utensils used to mix the feed
- During the preparation of the enteral diet delivery system
- During storage, i.e. if storage conditions are inappropriate
- From the hands of healthcare professionals handling the feed
- The environment, e.g. dust and air
- The administration set (reservoir, giving set, enteral tube)

both feed and delivery system preparation. Recent evidence has shown that ascending infection of the diet container from the enteral tube via the giving set can occur.[12] It is essential that feeding reservoirs and giving sets are changed every 24 hours.

Bolus feeding of an enteral diet produces an increased incidence of side effects including diarrhoea and bloating.[12] Continuous pump controlled feeding is recommended[12] with feeding regimens designed to meet the individual needs of the patient. The dilution of a feed or a reduction in the amount of feed volume administered has not been shown to reduce gastrointestinal side effects when enteral nutrition is commenced. Full-strength, full-volume diet should therefore be given as this does not limit dietary intake. Blockage of a feeding tube with feed will require tube replacement. Therefore, it is important that all tubes are flushed through with sterile water using an appropriately sized sterile syringe on a regular basis (a minimum of twice daily). The use of the guidewire to unblock a tube should be avoided. This could cause injury to the patient and perforation to the tube.

To help reduce the possibility of regurgitation and aspiration of feed, sitting the patient at 45° during the administration of a feed is recommended.[12] Between 2 and 2.5 litres is normally prescribed to an adult patient on a daily basis (provided the patient has no metabolic or fluid balance problems). Gastric aspirations should be taken 2–3 hourly during the initial 24 hours following the commencement of an enteral infusion. This is to ensure that the feed is being tolerated.

It is important that an accurate record of the fluid intake is kept. The patient's weight should also be recorded regularly. A weight gain of 1–2 kg per week suggests that an adequate diet is being provided. Biochemical and haematological parameters also need to be measured regularly.

References

1. Holmes, S. The aetiology of malnutrition in hospital. *Professional Nurse Study Supplement* 1998; 13(6): 55–58.

2. Rutishauser, S. *Physiology and Anatomy. A basis for nursing and healthcare.* 1994; Edinburgh: Churchill Livingstone.

3. Naber, T.H.J., Schermer, T., Bree, A. Prevalence of malnutrition in non-surgical hospitalised populations and its associations with disease complications. *American Journal of Clinical Nutrition* 1997; 60: 1232–1239.

4. Grindel, C.G., Costello, M.C. Nutrition screening: an essential assessment parameter. *Medical and Surgical Nursing* 1996; 5(3): 145–156.

5. Bristrian, B.R., Blackburn, G.L., Hallowell, E., Heddle, R. Protein status of general surgical patients. *Journal of the American Medical Association* 1974; 230(6): 858–860.

6. Bristrian, B.R., Blackburn, G.L., Vitale, J. *et al*. Prevalence of malnutrition in general medical patients. *Journal of the American Medical Association* 1976; 235: 1567–1570.

7. Hill, G.L., Pickford, I. Young, C.A. *et al*. Malnutrition in surgical patients. *Lancet* 1977; 1: 689–692.

8. McWhirter, J.P., Pennington, C.R. The incidence and recognition of malnutrition in hospitals. *British Medical Journal* 1994; 308: 945–948.

9. Rolando, H.R., Buckmire, M.A. Enteral nutrition in the surgical patient. In Payne-James, J., Grimble, G., Silk, D. (eds), *Artificial Nutrition Support in Clinical Practice* 1995; London: Edward Arnold.

10. McLaren, S. Nutritional Screening and Assessment. *Proffessional Nurse Study Supplement.* 1998; 13(6): 59–514.

11. Klein, S., Kinney, J., Jeejeebhoy, K. *et al*. Nutrition support in clinical practice: a review of published data and recommendations for future research directions. *Journal of Parenteral and Enteral Nutrition* 1997; 21: 133–156.

12. Payne-James, J. Enteral nutrition: tubes and techniques of delivery. In Payne-James, J., Grimble, G., Silk, D. (eds), *Artificial Nutrition Support in Clinical Practice* 1995; London: Edward Arnold.

Review questions

1. Label the following structures on the figure below: oesophagus, stomach, duodenum, jejunum, ileum, ascending colon, transverse colon, descending colon, sigmoid colon, rectum, anal canal.

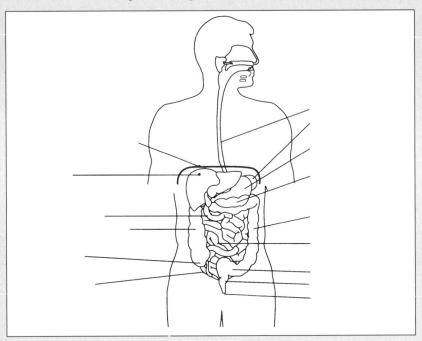

2. What is the major type of movement in the small intestine?

3. What structure prevents the regurgitation of food from the stomach back into the oesophagus?

4. What structure separates the stomach and the duodenum?

5. Name the different areas of the small intestine.

6. What is the major role of the small intestine?

7. What is the name of the movement only seen in the large intestine?

8. Which of the following are true?

    (a) 500 ml food material enters the caecum daily

    (b) Haustra are found in the small intestine

    (c) Absorption of nutrients occurs in the large intestine

    (d) Sodium, chloride and water are absorbed in the large intestine

9. Is it true to say that the longer food residue remains in the large intestine, the greater the quantity of water absorbed?

10. What is meant by nutritional screening?

11. List the different routes of enteral feeding.

12. How is the position of a FBT confirmed?

13. When should an X-ray be used to confirm the position of a FBT?

14. Which is the most common complication that causes an interruption of enteral feeding regimens?

15. When would jejunal or duodenal feeding be considered?

16. When should the guide-wire of a FBT never be used?

17. When would a PEG be used?

18. How frequently should feeding reservoirs and giving sets be changed?

19. Following the commencement of enteral feeding what action should be undertaken to ensure that the feed is being tolerated?

Review questions – answers

1.

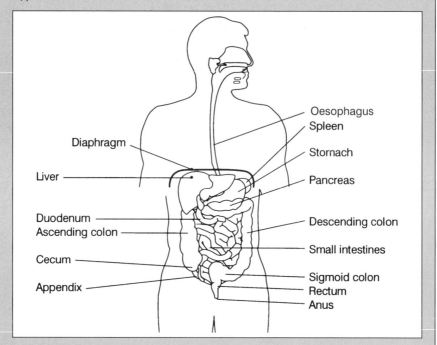

2. Segmentation

3. Oesophageal sphincter

4. Pyloric canal encased by the pyloric sphincter

5. Duodenum, jejunum, ileum

6. Nutrient absorption

7. Mass movement

8. a and d are true

9. Yes

10. A tool that enables a practitioner to identify patients at risk of malnutrition and those already malnourished

11. Nasoduodenal tube, nasogastric tube, gastrostomy tube, jejunostomy tube, oesophagostomy tube

12. Syringe aspiration of gastric contents (pH < 3)

13. When auscultation and gastric aspiration has been unsuccessful. In patients with altered consciousness levels, altered cough or gag reflex, and in mechanically ventilated patients

14. Unplanned removal by patients and staff

15. When there is a risk of regurgitation of feed or pulmonary aspiration

16. When the tube is in the patient

17. Long-term feeding, i.e. more than 3–4 weeks

18. Every 24 hours

19. Gastric aspiration 2–3 hourly

7

SUTURING

The suturing of simple lacerations of the skin, resulting from soft tissue injury, is an area of practice in which nursing staff are increasingly becoming involved. To undertake this practice safely and effectively, and to avoid problems such as scarring and infection, the knowledge and principles upon which this practice is based must be fully understood. The anatomy and physiology of the skin and the physiology of wound healing is presented below. This knowledge is then applied to the procedure for suturing.

APPLIED ANATOMY AND PHYSIOLOGY OF THE SKIN

The skin is the largest of the body's organs. It has a vast surface area, which spans about 2 m² and accounts for about 16% of an individual's total body weight.

The skin (**Figure 7.1**) is composed of two major layers of tissue; the outer **epidermis** and the inner **dermis.** It also has accessory structures including hair, nails, sweat glands and sebaceous glands. These structures, although in the dermis, protrude through the epidermis to the skin surface.

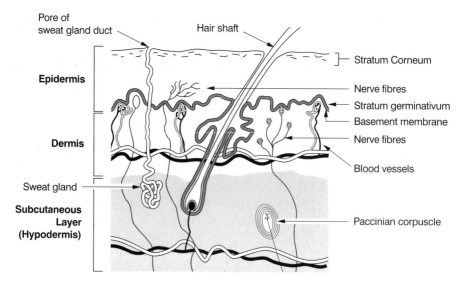

Figure 7.1 – The structure of the skin

The skin's functions include:

- Protection of underlying organs and tissues

- Excretion of waste products, salts and water

- Maintenance of normal body temperature

- Storage of nutrients

- Detection of stimuli such as temperature, and the relay of this information to the nervous system.[1]

Epidermis

The skin is persistently subjected to mechanical injury. The epidermis provides protection, and also prevents microorganisms from entering the body. It is comprised of a number of layers. The innermost layer of the epidermis is the **stratum germinativum**, and the outermost layer, the **stratum corneum**. The stratum germinativum is attached to a basement membrane, which separates the dermis from the epidermis.

The stratum germinativum is composed of many germinative or basal cells, the division of which replaces the cells shed at the epithelial surface. As these germinative cells move towards the skin's surface, their structure and activity changes. While still at the basal layer they begin forming the protein keratin. Its formation is continued as the cells move towards the skin's surface. Eventually, as the cells reach the stratum corneum, about 15–30 days later, they are like flattened bags of protein, and their intracellular organelles have disappeared.

Before they are lost from the stratum corneum, these cells remain in this layer for a further 2 weeks. This provides the underlying tissue with a protective barrier of cells, which although dead is exceedingly durable. The stratum corneum is the major barrier to the loss of water from the body. It has two actions that restrain the movement of water and limit the loss of water from the skin's surface. First, the matrix in which the cells of the stratum corneum are embedded is rich in lipid. This substance is almost impenetrable to water and, therefore, makes it extremely difficult for water molecules to move out of the epidermal cell. Second, protein inside the epidermal cells attracts and holds on to water molecules. As a consequence of these actions the surface of the skin is, therefore, normally dry, with very little water lost and so is an unsuitable place for the growth of many microorganisms. Although water-resistant, the stratum corneum is not waterproof. Interstitial fluid gradually penetrates this layer of tissue to be evaporated from the surface into the surrounding air. About 500 ml is lost from the body each day in this way.

Dermis

The dermis is comprised of a network of two types of protein: collagen and elastin. Collagen fibres provide strength to the skin; elastin gives the skin its flexibility. The dermis is also comprised of a network of blood vessels and other structures including sweat glands, which are all over the skin and secrete a dilute salt solution onto the skin's surface; sebaceous glands, found everywhere in the body except non-hairy areas, and secrete **sebum** that contains a mixture of lipids; sensory receptors; and defence cells.

There are variations in the structure of the skin in relation to age, environment and ethnic origin. The skin also varies between different parts of the body. For example, non-hairy (glabrous) skin, e.g. on the palms of hands and the soles of feet, has an extremely thick epidermis and numerous sensory receptors. The skin with hair follicles (hairy skin), e.g. on the scalp, has a thin epidermis and many sebaceous glands.

Physiology of wound healing

The skin protects against environmental hazards. During wounding, there is a breakdown in these protective functions. For example, microorganisms can enter the deeper tissues of the body and cause infection. In burn injuries, large areas of the skin's surface may be damaged to such an extent that fluid loss may become life-threatening.

Wounds can be classified by the layers of tissue involved. In superficial wounds, only the epidermis is effected. In partial-thickness wounds, injury extends as far as the dermis. Wounds that involve the subcutaneous fat or deeper layers are classified as full-thickness wounds. Several causes of wounding have been identified and described as those arising through:

- Trauma, i.e. mechanical, chemical or physical
- Surgery
- Ischaemia, e.g. arterial leg ulcer
- Pressure, e.g. pressure sore[2]

Suturing closes incision wounds. This method of wound closure eliminates dead space in the tissue, realigns tissue planes, and opposes and holds the skin edges until they have healed and no longer need artificial support. Healing takes place by primary intention and is accomplished within several days. However, in wounds caused by trauma where there is tissue loss and the wound edges are not opposed, the formation of new tissue is essential. This new tissue fills the wound and is then covered by epithelium. This is called healing by secondary intention and can take weeks or months.

Regardless of the nature of the tissue damage, the process of healing occurs in three overlapping phases:

- Inflammation
- Proliferation
- Maturation

Inflammation

Following tissue damage, bleeding generally occurs. A network of molecules, produced by **fibrinogen**, bring the wound edges in loose approximation. Fibrin (an insoluble protein that forms the basic framework of a blood clot) and other proteins dry at the surface and a scab is formed. This prevents further fluid loss and bacterial invasion. Meanwhile, serum proteins and white cells are leaked from blood vessels surrounding the wound. This accumulation of fluid in the tissue gives rise to the signs of inflammation, i.e. swelling, heat, redness and pain, and occurs within minutes of the injury. Following this, **neutrophils** and **macrophages** move into the damaged tissue to remove debris and ingest bacteria.

Proliferation

Following the inflammatory phase, tissue proliferation takes place. This phase involves:

- Formation of a network of new blood vessels in a collagen rich matrix, i.e. granulation, and the appearance of strands of collagen in the body of the wound
- Contraction of the wound, which minimizes its size
- Epithelialization, which involves the epithelial cells on the wound surface turning down over the edge of the underlying dermis and growing under the dried scab (**Figure 7.2**)

Maturation

During the final stage of healing the wound becomes less vascularized as there is a reduction in the need to bring blood cells to the wound site. The wound is also strengthened by the rearrangement of collagen fibres and the scar tissue is gradually remodelled, becoming comparable with normal tissue.

WOUND ASSESSMENT

Good wound management requires an accurate assessment so that the best possible conditions for healing can be provided. **Table 7.1** describes the areas to be included in a wound assessment.[3]

Wound closure material

Wound closure materials are available in many sizes and materials to accommodate the different requirements of the patient. The most appropriate suture material and needle must be selected to achieve the best outcome. The suture materials available can be divided into two main groups:

- Absorbable material
- Non-absorbable material

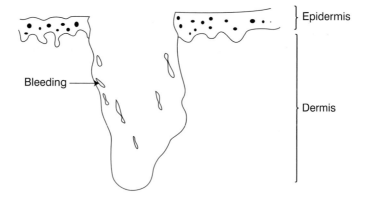

Bleeding at injury site immediately following injury

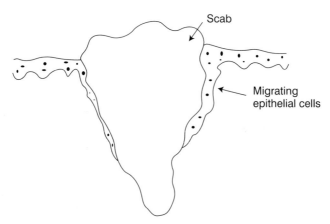

A scab has formed after several hours + epithelial cells on
wound surface are turning down over the edges of the
underlying dermis + growing under the dried scab

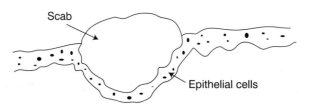

Epithelial cells have migrated and now cover the full area
beneath the scab

Figure 7.2 – The stages in skin regeneration following injury

Table 7.1 – *The areas covered in a wound assessment[3]*

Cause of injury
Did the injury involve a stab wound or was crushing, torsion or shearing applied?
For a penetrating injury, what was the instrument that caused the injury?
Did a blunt or sharp object cause the injury?
Was the instrument clean?
Examination
What is the position and size of the wound?
Is there any tissue loss?
Is deeper structure involvement suspected? (Formal wound exploration under local anaesthetic may be necessary to assess the full extent of the damage).
Have tendons been damaged or is damage suspected?
Is sensation around and distal to the wound normal?
Are any foreign bodies detectable or suspected? (An X-ray should be requested for all glass-related injuries.)
What was the time of injury?
Are any other injuries present?
What is the degree of pain experienced by the patient?
General health of the patient
What is the general state of the patient's health? Diabetic patients and those taking anticoagulant or steroid therapy may have delayed wound healing.
Has the patient any known allergies to the drugs, dressings and antiseptics likely to be used?
Has the patient recently had a tetanus injection? They should be treated according to the guidelines issued by the Joint Committee on Vaccination and Immunisation.[4]

Non-absorbable sutures are gentler on the tissue, only cause infrequent reaction or rejection and are widely used for skin closure.[3] Monofilament nylon is non-absorbable, consisting of a single, strong strand of nylon that gives strength to the wound until it has healed. Silk, also non-absorbable, is braided and although easy to use provides a large surface area for invasion by micro-organisms.[3]

Absorbable materials are most frequently used for suturing deeper layers of tissue. Tissue enzymes eventually break down these materials. Therefore, it is important to ensure that these materials will retain tensile strength for the duration of wound healing.[3] These types of sutures are also useful for patients who may not attend a follow-up appointment or, for those who might forget they have sutures.[3]

Following the selection of suture material, the size of suture, and size and type of needle must be identified. The suture material diameter is denoted numerically. The smaller the number, the larger the suture. The most frequently used sizes for simple, small wounds range from 3/0 (large) to 6/0[5] (fine). Recommended adult sizes should be reduced by one size when suturing children's wounds.[5] Different suturing techniques exist to meet the specific needs of the patient. The most simple and versatile method of skin closure is interrupted sutures. This method is used to close the majority of small fresh wounds.[3] Interrupted sutures have several advantages, including:

- Insertion of sutures is easier than with continuous suturing

- An incorrectly placed suture can easily be replaced

- In wounds where a cosmetic effect is paramount, e.g. facial wounds, or where the drainage of pus is necessary, alternate sutures can be removed

- Removal of the sutures is less painful for the patient

- Accurate wound edge alignment is more likely to be achieved and the cosmetic effect is normally good.[5]

There are other methods of wound closure, including the use of tissue adhesives, metal skin staples and adhesive tape strips. Adhesive paper tapes or tissue adhesives may be more suitable for wounds affecting fragile skin, as these wounds can tear easily and become necrotic if interrupted suturing is used.[6]

ANAESTHESIA

Formal wound exploration under local anaesthetic may be necessary, before suturing, to assess the full extent of the injury. Any foreign bodies must be removed. It is important to make sure that adequate local anaesthesia is administered to the patient before the wound cleansing and suturing procedures. Using a small sterile needle to apply pinprick sensations to the area surrounding the wound can ensure this.[5]

Lignocaine is the most widely used local anaesthetic. Its action is rapid, occurring within 3–5 minutes, the duration of its action being about 1.0–1.5 hours. When administered at the desired site of action, lignocaine penetrates the nerve axon and causes a reversible 'block' of conduction along the nerve fibres to produce a loss of sensation and a loss of muscle activity. The inhibition of nerve conduction persists until the drug diffuses and enters the circulation for subsequent metabolism and excretion.

Care must be taken not to exceed the maximum dosage of lignocaine when anaesthetising a wound. Dosage is dependent upon body weight (**Table 7.2**). In particular, care must be taken in infants and young children. The systemic side-effects of lignocaine due to excessive application and increased absorption include: convulsions, paraesthesia, nervousness, tremors, hypotension and bradycardia.[7]

Lignocaine can be diluted with an equal amount of normal saline, in order that a small concentration can be used to infiltrate the whole wound. Depending on hospital protocol, it may be recommended that nurses are only responsible for administering half the maximum amount of lignocaine, after which medical advice should be sought.

Lignocaine can be injected into the subcutaneous tissue via the wound space. If the wound is contaminated the needle should be inserted through the skin on either side of the wound.[3] Resistance may be felt during injection of the fluid, in which case the needle should be inserted more deeply into the subcutaneous tissue.[3] Combined lignocaine and adrenaline preparations should not be used without a prescription. Although this preparation causes an increase in the duration of block in nerve conduction, adrenaline causes peripheral vaso-constriction. It is contraindicated for infiltration of areas with end arteries (e.g. fingers, toes, ears, nose) as ischaemia may occur resulting in tissue death.[8]

WOUND CLEANSING

Current thinking suggests that the best method is to irrigate the wound under pressure, with normal saline or sterile water.[9] Contaminated wounds should be treated with a broad spectrum antiseptic solution.

Table 7.2 – Maximum dosages of lignocaine to be administered when anaesthetizing a wound[3]

Weight (kg)	Maximum dose (mg)	Volume of 1% solution (ml)	Volume of 2% solution (ml)
5	5–15	0.5–1.5	0.25–0.75
10	10–30	1–3	0.5–1.5
20	20–60	2–6	1.0–3.0
30	30–90	3–9	1.5–4.5
50 (adult)	150	15	7.5
70 (adult)	210	21	10.5

Suturing the wound

Following anaesthetising and cleansing of the wound, interrupted sutures can be inserted. Suturing should generally commence at the centre of linear wounds, as this will maintain wound edge alignment.

The following need to be considered:[3,5]

- The insertion of the needle should not be closer than 5 mm from the wound edge. This prevents the sutures from being pulled out and allows the wound edges to evert. This will result in a flattened scar and a good cosmetic effect.

- The needle should be inserted at a 90° angle. This will allow a full -thickness 'bite' and prevent the skin edges inverting and blood collecting in the wound base.

- Needle insertion should be undertaken separately into each side of the wound.

- Suture knots should be on the same side of the wound and cut free from the suture before the next insertion.

- Sufficient space should be left between each suture for the escape of wound exudate.

- Too few sutures will cause the wound to gape and increase the risk off infection and scarring. Too many sutures will cause tension and reduce blood flow, possible necrosis, delayed healing and a poor cosmetic effect.

- Non-adherent dressings should be used until the sutures are removed. Some wounds eg. scalp and facial wounds may not require a dressing.

It is important that on discharge home the patient or carer is provided with enough information to care for the wound. This should include information on dressing changes, symptoms and signs of wound healing problems, and follow-up appointments.

Suture removal is dependent upon the period that the wound edges require support. This must be balanced by the fact that the earlier the sutures are removed, the better the end cosmetic result.

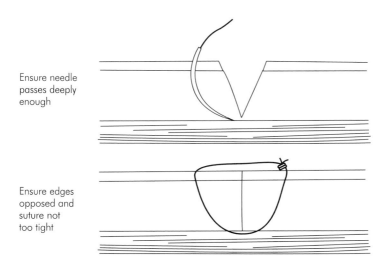

Ensure needle passes deeply enough

Ensure edges opposed and suture not too tight

Figure 7.3 – Correct wound suturing technique

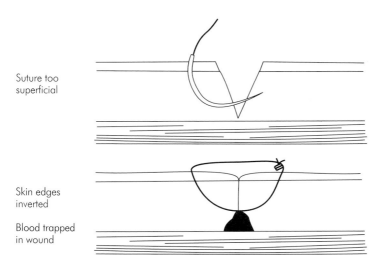

Suture too superficial

Skin edges inverted

Blood trapped in wound

Figure 7.4 – Incorrect wound suturing techniques

References

1. Martini, F.H. *Fundamentals of Anatomy and Physiology* (4th edition). 1998; Englewood Cliffs: Prentice Hall.

2. Dealey, C. *The Care of Wounds*. 1994; Oxford: Blackwell Scientific.

3. Jay, R. Suturing in A&E. *Professional Nurse* 1999; 14: 412–415.

4. Joint Committee on Vaccination and Immunisation *Immunisation against Diseases*. 1996; London: HMSO.

5. Castille, K. Suturing. *Nursing Standard* 1998; 12(41): 41–48.

6. Castille, K. Suturing. *Emergency Nurse* 1997; 5: 29–34.

7. Courtenay, M., Butler, M. *Nurse Prescribing: Principles and Practice*. 1999; London: Greenwich Medical Media.

8. Clarke, J.B., Queener, S.F., Karb, V. *Pharmacological Basis of Nursing Practice* (5th edition). 1997. St Louis: C.V. Mosby.

9. Miller, M., Dyson, M. *Principles of Wound Care*. 1996; London: Macmillan.

Review questions

1. Approximately how many skin scales drop from one's body in 1 min?

2. What are the two major layers of the skin?

3. Skin cells contain the protein keratin. In what other structures can it be found?

4. List four functions of the skin.

5. Is it true that when basal cells reach the skin surface they are dead?

6. Is it true that these basal cells are full of fat?

7. How does the stratum corneum limit the loss of water from the skin's surface?

8. What structures make up the dermis?

9. Identify the tissue involved in superficial wounds, partial-thickness wounds and full-thickness wounds?

10. What does healing by primary intention mean?

11. What does healing by secondary intention mean?

12. What are the phases of wound healing?

13. Identify the areas that would be included in a wound assessment.

14. What are the side-effects of lignocaine if given in too larger dose?

15. What effect can adrenaline cause if combined with lignocaine and injected into areas of the body with end arteries?

16. When are absorbable materials commonly used?

Review questions – answers

1. 35 000

2. Epidermis and dermis

3. Hair and nails

4. Protection of organs and tissue, excretion of salt, water and urea, temperature regulation, maintenance of body shape, protection of excessive water loss from the body

5. Yes

6. No, they are full of protein

7. The cells of the stratum corneum are embedded in a lipid-rich matrix. This makes it very difficult for water to move out of the epidermal cells. Second, the protein inside the epidermal cells attracts and holds onto water molecules

8. Proteins, collagen, elastin, blood vessels, sebaceous glands, sensory receptors, defence cells, sweat glands.

9. Superficial wounds involve the epidermis, partial-thickness wounds involve the dermis, full-thickness wounds involve subcutaneous fat or deeper layers

10. There is no new tissue formation

11. There is new tissue formation

12. Inflammation, proliferation, maturation

13. See **Table 7.1**

14. Convulsions, paraesthesia, nervousness, tremors, hypotension and bradycardia

15. Vasoconstriction

16. When suturing deeper layers of tissue

8

MALE CATHETERIZATION

Urinary catheterization is an integral part of the care of many patients. For patients nursed at home, the prevalence of urinary catheterization is 4%.[1] In hospital, 10% of patients are catheterized at some time during admission.[2] It is evident from the literature that the issue of female nurses catheterizing male patients is a controversial subject.[3-6] Historically, male catheterization has been the responsibility of male nurses and doctors. The reasons for this are unclear. However, it is recognized by *The Scope of Professional Practice*[7] that practice 'must be sensitive, relevant and responsive to the needs of individual patients and have the capacity to adjust'. The principles underpinning this document, therefore, facilitate the incorporation of the skills of male catheterization into everyday nursing practice, male patients having the opportunity of receiving holistic rather than fragmented care. This chapter commences with a description of the anatomy and physiology of the urinary system, followed by an examination of the procedure for male catheterization. Finally, the basic principles of infection control and their application to male catheterization are discussed.

APPLIED ANATOMY AND PHYSIOLOGY

Urinary system

The primary function of the urinary system (**Figure 8.1**) is the elimination of water-soluble substances. Urine, containing electrolytes, water and nutrients, is produced by the kidneys. It passes through the paired ureters to the bladder, where it is stored until excreted. During excretion, or **micturition**, urine is forced from the bladder into the urethra, and then out of the body.

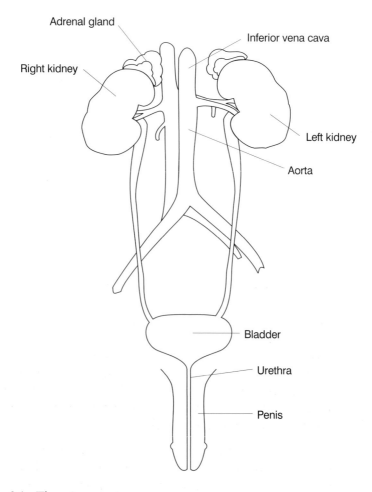

Figure 8.1 – The urinary system

Kidneys

The kidneys are responsible for the continuous formation of urine. They are at the back of the abdomen on either side of the vertebral column. Each weighs about 140 g and is the shape of a kidney bean. In adults, the kidney is about 10 cm in length, 5 cm in width and is 3 cm thick. Each kidney is made up of about 1 million tiny tubes called **nephrons**. These are the functional units of the kidney and are responsible for urine production. Each nephron has a rich blood supply. The kidney receives close to 25% of the total cardiac output and filters about 150 litres of fluid from the blood plasma each day. Only about 1–2 litres of this fluid is excreted. The remainder is returned to the blood.

Ureters

The ureters are about 30 cm in length and extend inferiorly from each kidney to the bladder. The ureter walls possess smooth muscle. Urine is forced towards the urinary bladder in spurts by peristaltic contractions of these muscles. The epithelial cells lining both the ureters and the bladder are highly impermeable to water. Therefore, there is no movement of fluid from these structures into the blood. The ureters enter the bladder at an oblique angle. During contraction of the bladder, the bladder walls compress the openings of the ureters and prevent the back flow of urine.

Bladder

The urinary bladder is a hollow muscular organ that stores urine temporarily. As urine flows into the bladder from the ureters it becomes distended. The bladder wall contains layers of longitudinal and circular smooth muscle. These layers form the **detrusor** muscle. Contraction of this muscle compresses the bladder and causes urine to be expelled into the urethra. The trigone is the triangular area near the mouth of the bladder through which both the ureters and the urethra pass (**Figure 8.2**). During contraction of the bladder, the trigone funnels urine into the urethra. The maximum volume of fluid that the bladder can hold varies, but without too much discomfort, it is normally about 0.5 litres.

The neck of the bladder, the area that surrounds the urethral opening, contains an internal urethral sphincter. The smooth muscle fibres of this sphincter involuntarily control the discharge of urine from the bladder. Below the bladder, the urethra passes through the urogenital diaphragm.

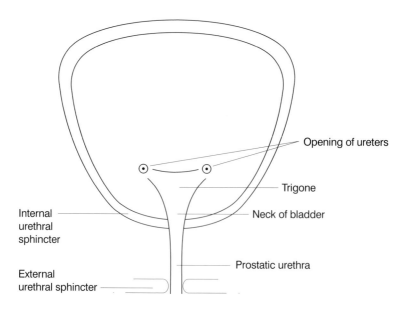

Figure 8.2 – The bladder

Urethra

The bladder is connected to the exterior surface of the body by the urethra. This structure is 3–5 cm long in the female and 18–20 cm long in the male. In the female, the external urethral opening is positioned near the anterior wall of the vagina. In the male, the urethra is divided into three sections (**Figure 8.3**):

- The prostatic urethra, which passes through the centre of the prostate gland.

- The membranous urethra, which penetrates the urogenital diaphragm.

- The penile urethra, which extends from the urogenital diaphragm to the tip of the penis.

As the urethra passes through the urogenital diaphragm, a circular band of voluntary skeletal muscle forms the external urethral sphincter. This sphincter is normally contracted, and escape of urine is prevented.

Micturition reflex

The process of urination is coordinated by the micturition reflex, which involves both involuntary and voluntary mechanisms. Involuntary control

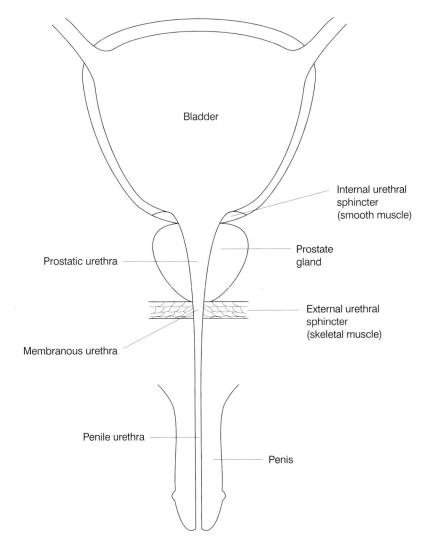

Bladder

Internal urethral
sphincter
(smooth muscle)

Prostate
gland

Prostatic urethra

External urethral
sphincter
(skeletal muscle)

Membranous urethra

Penile urethra

Penis

Figure 8.3 – The male urethra

is by stretch receptors in the wall of the bladder, which become stimulated as the bladder distends. The desire to urinate normally occurs when the bladder contains about 500 ml urine. Once these receptors have become stimulated, the smooth muscle of the bladder contracts. These contractions elevate fluid pressure within the bladder. If both external and internal urethral sphincters are relaxed, urine is ejected. The external sphincter is relaxed under voluntary control. If the external sphincter relaxes then so does the internal sphincter. If the external sphincter does not relax, for example if it is impossible to visit a toilet, the internal sphincter does not open and the bladder is prevented from emptying. The bladder then relaxes. This cycle commences again with further increase in fluid volume in the bladder. This increase in volume leads to an increase in stretch receptor stimulation, making the sensation more acute. If the volume of urine is greater than 500 ml, the micturition reflex may generate sufficient pressure so that the internal urethral sphincter is forced to open. Relaxation of the external sphinter occurs followed by urination, despite possible inconvenience.

The pressure exerted by simultaneous contraction of the abdominal muscles also assists bladder emptying. However, the increases in abdominal pressure when sneezing or coughing can also provoke a loss of urine (**stress incontinence**). This tends to be more common in women than men.

Urinary catheterization

Urinary catheterization is the insertion of a catheter into the bladder via the urethral orifice. Urinary catheters are used for many reasons, including:

- To re-establish urine flow in urinary retention.

- To provide a channel for the drainage of urine when micturition is impaired.

- To maintain a dry environment in urinary incontinence when all other forms of nursing intervention have failed.

- To empty the bladder pre-operatively.

- To monitor fluid balance in a seriously ill patient.

- To facilitate bladder irrigation procedures.[8]

Procedure for male catheterization

It is important that before catheterization the patient's general condition is noted and the bladder is palpated. If it is anticipated that there will be complications, a doctor can then be informed. For example, a very distended bladder should be drained by slow decompression under medical supervision.[4] The equipment for urinary catheterization should then be assembled. This equipment should include:

- Sterile gloves

- Sterile catheterization pack or dressing pack

- Sterile water-based solution for cleansing the genitalia

- If required, sterile anaesthetic gel, or water-soluble lubricant

- Sterile receiver

- Sterile catheter

- Equipment for catheter balloon inflation, e.g. sterile water, needle and syringe

- Sterile closed drainage system

- Hypo-allergenic tape

- Labelled, sterile specimen container, completed laboratory form, plastic speciment bag for transportation

- Receptacle for soiled disposables[8]

Following assembly of catheterization equipment, the external **urethral meatus** must be cleansed using the sterile water-based solution. This procedure should be undertaken wearing sterile gloves, the penis being held with a gauze swab. Identification of the urethral meatus should not be a problem if the **prepuce** (foreskin) is easily retracted or absent. However, if the prepuce cannot be retracted over the glans of the penis (**phimosis**), difficulties may be encountered. If this situation arises, it is important that the prepuce is not forced. This can result in pain, trauma and **paraphimosis** (inflammation of the foreskin in a retracted position and the foreskin unable to be drawn back over the glans).[4] If phimosis is present, local anaesthetic gel can be instilled to dilate the prepuce.[4] This will desensitize the glans, allow the nurse to cleanse the meatus and allow the instillation of further gel into the urethra to anaesthetize it. Other conditions that can give rise to difficulties when identifying the urethral meatus are **hypospadias** (an abnormal urethral opening on the ventral surface of the shaft of the penis) and **epispadias** (an abnormal location of the urethral opening on the dorsal midline of the shaft of the penis).[4]

Following instillation of the gel into the urethra, 3 or 4 minutes should be allowed for local anaesthesia to take place. Straightening the penis should then extend the peno-scrotal flexure and the appropriate catheter should be gently introduced into the external meatus.

Selection of urinary catheters

The selection of the catheter material should be based on the needs of the patient, i.e. the intended duration of catheterization (**Table 8.1** has some guidance for catheter selection). Unless otherwise indicated, the use of size 12–16Ch is advised for men.[9] The use of large gauge catheters (> 16Ch) is associated with pressure necrosis,[10] bypassing of urine and discomfort.[11] Furthermore, the use of catheters with balloon sizes greater than 10 ml are associated with the ulceration of the bladder or urethral wall,[12] and leakage of urine.[13] Therefore, a larger balloon size should not be used, unless otherwise indicated, such as post-prostatectomy.

It is important that undue force is not used when introducing the catheter as this may cause urethral trauma.[14,15] However, following insertion of the catheter, some resistance may be felt at the external sphincter (about 15–20 cm after insertion). Asking the patient to cough or 'bear down' as though trying to pass urine may help to overcome this.[4] In the older male patient, greater pressure may be required to pass the catheter through the section of the urethra surrounded by the prostate gland. Nevertheless, if more than slight discomfort is felt by the patient, advice should be sought. Once it is evident that urine is flowing from the catheter, the catheter should be inserted a further 2–3 cm to ensure the balloon is in the bladder.[4] The

Table 8.1 – Types of catheter[30]

Catheter type	Material	Use
Foley two way: A channel for urine drainage, a channel for inflation of balloon.	Various (as described below)	Short, medium or long term drainage
Foley three way: A channel for urine, one for irrigation fluid, and one for inflation of balloon.	Latex Teflon Silicone Plastic	For continuous irrigation. Potential for infection minimal as need to break system is reduced.
Non-balloon (Nelaton) or intermittent catheter (one channel) or Scotts.	PVC Plastics	Intermittent emptying of bladder. Instil solutions into bladder.

balloon should then be inflated according to the instructions of the manufacturer, and the catheter withdrawn slowly until slight resistance is felt. The patient's prepuce should be replaced in its original position, and a suitable drainage system attached to the catheter. It is important that the catheter type, size, batch number and expiry date are recorded in the patient's notes, together with the date the catheter needs changing. Any changes in the patient's condition following the procedure should be reported. Post-catheterization haemorrhage rarely occurs providing the procedure is undertaken gently. If haemorrhage does occur, the volume of blood lost should be recorded and advice sought.

Importance of asepsis during catheterization

The urinary tract is one of the most frequently affected sites of nosocomial infection. The National Prevalence Study[16] reported that 30% of all nosocomial infections are urinary tract infections. These infections occurred mainly in those patients who were catheterized. The bladder has little defence against invading pathogens and, therefore, an infection may develop from only a small inoculum of bacteria.[17] The presence of an indwelling urethral catheter increases this risk. It has been identified[18] that 44% of patients develop significant bacteriuria within 72 hours of catheterization, rising to 90% 17 days later.

Gram-negative bacilli and *Staphylococcus epidermis* are the microorganisms primarily responsible for urinary tract infections.[19] The virulence of some of these microorganisms is enhanced by pili (minute hair-like processes) that allow them to attach themselves to the mucosal surface of the urinary tract. The bacteria responsible for urinary tract infections are frequently resistant to antibiotics.[19]

There is some debate within the literature on the source of the pathogens causing urinary tract infection in individuals who are catheterized. It has been suggested[20] that if patients are catheterized for less than 7 days bacteria are likely to enter the drainage system from either the drainage tap or following disconnection of the system. However, as the period during which the patient is catheterized increases, bacteria are more likely to enter the bladder alongside the catheter and along the wall of the urethra (peri-urethral space).[20] It has also been suggested that migration of infection from a contaminated urinary bag is another major route.[21] The hands of practitioners and patients have also been associated with catheter-related infection.[22] Strict hand hygiene is, therefore, essential by both nurses and patients. **Figure 8.4** highlights the possible portals of entry of bacteria into the urinary tract via a closed drainage system.

Secondary complications associated with urinary tract infection

Secondary complications associated with urinary tract infection include encrustation and blockage, bypassing, tissue damage and patient discomfort.[11,12] Encrustation affects 16–28% of catheterized patients.[19] Microorganisms such as *Proteus*, *Klebsiella* and *Pseudomonas* cause an increase in urine alkalinity. This encourages the process of encrustation causing the precipitation of various salts from the urine. Blockage to the catheter occurs when the catheter becomes encrusted and the eye of the catheter becomes occluded. Leakage then occurs around the outside of the catheter following blockage. The presence of a biofilm on the catheter surface also increases the risk of encrustation.[23] A biofilm is the collection of microorganisms and

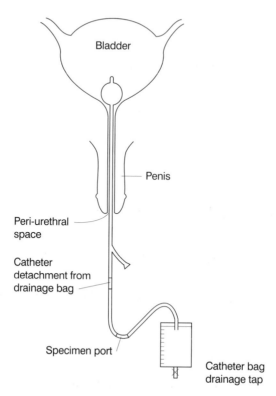

Figure 8.4 – Portals of entry into the closed drainage system

their products on a solid surface.[24] Bacteria within this film are protected from antimicrobial drugs and the body's natural defence mechanisms.

It has been suggested that by observing and recording the time a catheter remains *in situ* before becoming blocked will reveal a pattern of 'catheter life'.[25] This will enable recatheterization before blockage occurs. The consumption of cranberry juice may also assist in prolonging catheter life by acidification of the urine and by the prevention of encrustation.[26]

The risk of infection is greater for patients with severe underlying illness. There is little doubt that urinary tract infection associated with catheterization contributes directly to morbidity and may result in patient mortality.[27,28] Clifford[29] suggested that between 40 000 and 50 000 patients develop septicaemia through ascending urinary tract infection each year in the UK. For about 500 of these, the consequences are fatal. Therefore, it is essential that before catheterization a careful assessment of the patient is undertaken to ensure that catheterization is in the best interest of the patient, and that alternative treatment methods would not be more suitable.

References

1. Roe, B. Catheters in the community. *Nursing Times* 1989; 85(36): 43–44.

2. Mulhal, A., Chapman, R.G., Crow, R.A. Bacteriuria during in-dwelling catheterisation. *Journal of Hospital Infection* 1988; 11: 235–262.

3. Pomfret, I. An unsuitable job for a woman. *Nursing Times* 1994; 90(22): 46–48.

4. Pomfret, I. Men only. *Nursing Times* 1993; 89(8): 55–58.

5. Pottle, B. Equal rites for men. *Nursing Times* 1992; 88(44): 74.

6. Fader, M. New thoughts on male catheterisation. *Nursing Times* 1996; 82(15): 64–66.

7. United Kingdom Central Council for Nursing, Midwifery, and Health Visiting *The Scope of Professional Practice.* 1992; London: UKCC.

8. Jamieson, E.M., McCall, J.M., Blythe, R., Whyte, L. *Clinical Nursing Practices.* 1997; London: Churchill Livingstone.

9. Roe, B. Catheter-associated urinary tract infections. A review. *Journal of Clinical Nursing* 1993; 2: 197–203.

10. Blandy, J.P. Urethral stricture. *Post Graduate Medical Journal* 1980; 56: 383–418.

11. Roe, B., Brocklehurst, J.C. Study of patients with in-dwelling catheters. *Journal of Advanced Nursing* 1987; 12(6): 713–718.

12. Getliffe, K. Informed choices for long term benefits. The management of catheters in continence care. *Professional Nurse* 1993; 9(2): 122–126.

13. Kennedy, A.P. *et al*. Factors related to the problems of long term catheterisation. *Journal of Advanced Nursing* 1983; 8: 207–212.

14. Burkitt, D.S., Randall, J. Catheterisation: urethral trauma. *Nursing Times* 1987; 83(43): 59–60, 63.

15. Royal College of Nursing Continence Care Forum *Guidelines on Male Catheterisation: The Role of the Nurse.* 1984; London: RCN.

16. Meers, P.D., Ayliffe, G.A.G., Emmerson, A.M. *et al*. Report of the National Survey of Infection in Hospitals. *Journal of Hospital Infection* 1981; 2: 23–28.

17. Stickler, D.J., Chawla, J.C. The role of antiseptics in the management of patients with long term indwelling bladder catheters. *Journal of Hospital Infection* 1987; 10: 219–228.

18. Crow, R., Chapman, R., Roe, B., Wilson, J. *Study of Patients with an In-dwelling Urinary Catheter and Related Nursing Practice.* 1986; Guildford: Nursing Practice Research Unit, University of Surrey.

19. Gould, D. Keeping on tract. *Nursing Times* 1994; 90(40): 58–64.

20. Nickel, J.C., Grant, S.K., Costerton, J.W. Catheters – associated bacteriuria, an experimental study. *Urology* 1985; 36: 369–375.

21. Maizels, M., Schaefer, A.J. Decreased incidence of bacteriuria – associated instillation of hydrogen peroxide into the urethral catheter. *Journal of Urology* 1980; 123: 841–845.

22. Sanderson, P.J., Weissler, S. Recovery of coliforms from the hands of nurses and patients: activities leading to contamination. *Journal of Hospital Infection* 1992; 21: 85–94.

23. Ramsey, J. Biofilm, bacteria, and bladder catheters – a clinical study. *British Journal of Urology* 1989; 64: 395–398.

24. Wilson, M. Infection control. *Professional Nurse Study Supplement* 1989; 13(5): S10–13.

25. Getliffe, K. Care of urinary catheters. *Nursing Standard* 1996; 11(11): 47–50.

26. Busuttil Leaver, R. Cranberry juice. *Professional Nurse* 1996; 11(8): 525–526.

27. Platt, R., Polk, B.F., Murdoch, B., Rosner, B. Reduction of mortality associated with nosocomial urinary tract infection. *Lancet* 1983; 893–897.

28. Kunin, C.M., Douthitt, S., Daning, J. *et al.* The association between the use of urinary catheters and morbidity and mortality among elderly patients in nursing homes. *American Journal of Epidemiology* 1992; 123: 291–301.

29. Clifford, C.M. Urinary tract infection; a brief selective review. *International Journal of Nursing Studies* 1982; 19: 213–222.

30. Mallet, J., Bailey, C. *The Royal Marsden NHS Trust Manual of Clinical Nursing Procedures* (4th edition). 1996; Oxford: Blackwell Science.

Review questions

1. Is the detrusor muscle a voluntary or involuntary muscle?

2. In what area of the bladder are the ureteric and urethral openings found?

3. When not micturating, is the urethra open or closed?

4. How is urine passed to the bladder via the kidney?

5. Of what types of muscle are the external and internal sphincters of the bladder composed?

6. How does one know when one wishes to void?

7. Consider a patient with an in-dwelling urinary catheter. Identify the possible sites whereby bacteria may enter the closed drainage system.

8. Identify five complications associated with male catheterization

9. What does the Charriere (Ch) or French Gauge (FG) of the catheter denote?

10. What is the most appropriate size of catheter to use for a male patient?

11. What problems can catheters with large lumens cause?

12. When may a large lumen catheter be justified?

13. What solution should be used to fill the catheter balloon?

14. Why may urine bypass a catheter?

15. Case study

Following a cystoscopy to investigate intermittent urethral dribbling, a male patient has been discharged from hospital. Upon return to the outpatient's clinic for a review of his treatment, the patient complains that the present system of incontinence pads he has been using is causing problems. Following discussion, it is decided that urethral catheterization is the most appropriate course of action.

- The catheter is to remain in situ for up to 3 months. Which catheter material is the most appropriate?

- Once the catheter has been inserted into the patient's bladder and urine is flowing, what step would one take next?

- Why is it important following the procedure to ensure that the patient's prepuce is placed back over the glans?

- Following catheterization of the patient, what details of the procedure should be documented?

- With which UKCC guidelines is this in accordance?

Review questions – answers

1. Involuntary

2. Trigone

3. Closed

4. Gravity and peristalsis

5. Internal – smooth muscle; external – striated muscle

6. Stretch receptors in the bladder wall are stimulated and these then send signals to the brain

7. On the tip of the catheter during insertion

   - During disconnection between the drainage bag and the catheter tubing

   - If the drainage bag was contaminated, microorganisms could migrate along the catheter tubing

   - From the space between the urethra and the outside of the catheter

8. Urinary tract infection, blockage, encrustation, bypassing, tissue damage

9. Gauge size

10. 12–16Ch

11. Pressure necrosis

12. Post-prostatectomy

13. Sterile water

14. When balloon sizes larger than 10 ml are used/Ch size to large

15.
   - Silicone-elastomer coated

   - Insert the catheter to the bifurcation to avoid inflating the balloon in the urethra

   - To prevent a paraphimosis

   - Catheter type, size, batch number and expiry date together with the date that the catheter needs changing

   - UKCC's standards for records and record-keeping (UKCC 1994)

Appendix 1

GLOSSARY OF TERMS

Absolute refractory period: For a certain period after an action potential begins, the cell membrane will not respond to another stimulus regardless of how strong the stimulus is. This is known as the absolute refractory period.

Action potential: The distinctive change in voltage between the inside and outside of neurones and muscle cells, initiated by a change in membrane permeability to sodium ions.

Anticoagulants: A substance that interferes with the clotting system and prevents or slows clotting.

Automaticity: Depolarisation to threshold spontaneously.

Biofilm: A collection of micro-organisms and their products on a solid surface.

Bolus: Compact mass.

Bradycardia: A slow heart rate.

Cardiac tamponade: The accumulation of fluid in the pericardial cavity causing compression of the heart.

Chyme: A mixture of food and digestive secretions in the stomach.

Collagen: A protein fibre present in connective tissue.

Depolarization: The movement of a transmembrane potential towards 0 mV.

Detrusor muscle: The longitudinal and circular smooth muscle in the bladder wall.

Diastole: The period during which the left ventricle relaxes following systole.

Ectopic pacemaker: When a conducting cell or ventricular muscle cell generates an action potential more rapidly than the SA or AV node.

Elastin: A fibre that provides elasticity to connective tissue.

Embolus: Fat globule, air bubble, or blood clot floating in the circulation.

Emulsion: A fluid formed by the suspension of one liquid in another.

Encrustation: Precipitation of salts from the urine, causing blockage of the urinary catheter.

Enzyme: A protein that accelerates a specific biochemical reaction.

Epispadias: An abnormal location of the urethral opening on the dorsal midline of the shaft of the penis.

Extravasion: The infusion of drugs or fluid into the tissues instead of the venous circulation.

Fibrinogen: A plasma protein.

Gap junction: A connection that links cells together allowing electrical coupling.

Graded potentials: Changes in transmembrane potential that cannot spread far from the site of stimulation.

Granulation: The new tissue formed in repair of wounds of soft tissue.

Haustra: Pouches in the wall of the large intestine.

Heart block: When the conduction pathway and normal heart rhythm are damaged.

Hypospadias: An abnormal urethral opening on the ventral surface of the shaft of the penis.

Inflammation: A defence mechanism characterised by swelling, heat, pain, and redness of the tissues.

Ion: A positive or negatively charged atom or molecule.

Ischaemia: An inadequate blood supply to an area of the body.

Keratin: The fibrous protein component of nails and hair.

Membrane channels: The channels enable ions to cross a cell membrane.

Mucosa: The inner lining of the digestive tract facing the digestive contents.

Mucus: A fluid that lubricates the respiratory, digestive, reproductive and urinary tracts.

Nephrons: The small tubes that make up the kidney.

Nosocomial infection: An infection that has its onset during hospitalisation.

Pacemaker cells: The cells of the SA node that control the rate of cardiac contraction.

Palpate: To examine by touching.

Paraphimosis: Inflammation of the foreskin in a retracted position, with the foreskin unable to be drawn back over the glans.

Peristalsis: Waves of smooth muscle contraction that drive material along a tube (e.g. the digestive tract).

pH: The concentration of hydrogen ions in a fluid, expressed in moles per litre.

Phimosis: When the prepuce cannot be retracted over the glans of the penis.

Pili: Minute hair-like processes. Found on micro-organisms.

Pneumothorax: Air in the pleural cavity.

Potential difference: A difference that exists when positive and negative ions are held apart.

Prepuce: Foreskin.

Primary intention healing: Wounds which can be closed by suturing and require only the formation of a small quantity of new tissue. This process is accomplished within several days.

Refractory period: For a certain period after an action potential begins, the cell membrane will not respond to another stimulus. This is called the refractory period.

Repolarization: When the cell membrane is in its resting state.

Resting potential: The transmembrane potential in an undisturbed cell.

Sebum: A wax like secretion coating the surface of hairs.

Secondary intention healing: Wounds in which there is tissue loss, and healing involves the formation of new tissue. This process can take weeks or months.

Segmentation: Movements seen in the small intestine, which mix digestive material with intestinal secretions.

Serosa: The serous membrane in the digestive tract.

Sphincter: A ring of muscle that, on contraction, closes an entrance or exit of an internal passageway.

Stratum corneum: The outermost layer of the epidermis.

Stratum germinativum: The innermost layer of the epidermis.

Stretch receptors: A sensory receptor that reacts when surrounding tissue is stretched.

Systole: The period of contraction of the left ventricle.

Tachycardia: A rapid heart rate.

Threshold: An action potential will commence at a certain transmembrane potential. This is known as threshold.

Thromboembolism: The blockage of a vessel by a blood clot.

Transmembrane potential: The potential difference across a cell membrane.

Transthoracic impedence (TTI): The resistance created by a structure in the thorax to an electrical current as it passes through the chest.

Vesicant fluids: Fluids that are irritant to tissues and lead to necrosis.

INDEX